Breaking Free from Asthma!

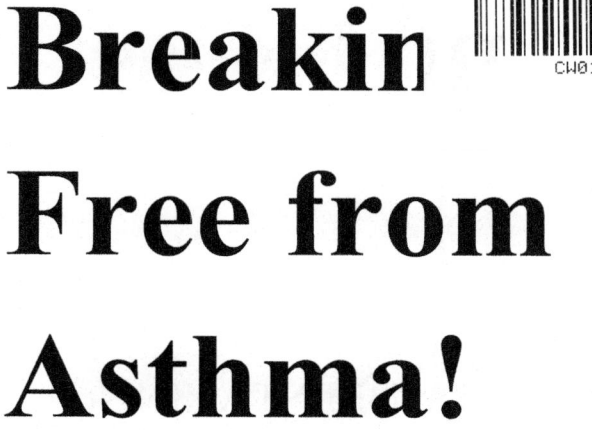

Your Essential Guide to Managing and Overcoming Respiratory Challenges

Louis Baker

CONTENTS OVERVIEW

FOREWARD

CHAPTER 1: UNDERSTANDING THE FUNDAMENTALS OF ASTHMA

CHAPTER 2: BUILDING YOUR HEALTHCARE SUPPORT TEAM

CHAPTER 3: MAXIMIZING YOUR DOCTOR VISITS

CHAPTER 4: ACHIEVING WELLNESS WITH ASTHMA

CHAPTER 5: LONG-TERM ASTHMA MANAGEMENT

CHAPTER 6: IDENTIFYING ASTHMA TRIGGERS

CHAPTER 7: INHALANT ALLERGIES AND THEIR IMPACT

CHAPTER 8: FOOD ALLERGIES AND ASTHMA

CHAPTER 9: MANAGING EXERCISE AND EMOTIONAL HEALTH

CHAPTER 10: ADDRESSING COEXISTING MEDICAL CONDITIONS

CHAPTER 11: ALLERGY TESTING AND IMMUNOTHERAPY

CHAPTER 12: COMPREHENSIVE GUIDE TO ASTHMA MEDICATIONS

CHAPTER 13: UNDERSTANDING ASTHMA CONTROLLER MEDICATIONS

CHAPTER 14: TREATING ASTHMA EPISODES EFFECTIVELY

CHAPTER 15: ASTHMA IN CHILDREN AND ADOLESCENTS

CHAPTER 16: ASTHMA MANAGEMENT DURING PREGNANCY

CHAPTER 17: ASTHMA CONCERNS IN OLDER ADULTS

CHAPTER 18: ADDITIONAL CONSIDERATIONS FOR ASTHMA

CHAPTER 19: ADVOCATING FOR YOURSELF AND OTHERS WITH ASTHMA

CHAPTER 20: TRUSTED RESOURCES FOR ASTHMA MANAGEMENT

CHAPTER 21: TIPS FOR TRAVELING WITH ASTHMA

CHAPTER 22: DISPELLING MYTHS ABOUT ASTHMA AND ALLERGIES

CHAPTER 23: STRATEGIES TO NAVIGATE THE SEPTEMBER ASTHMA PEAK

LAST CHAPTER: COMMON QUESTIONS ASKED BY PATIENTS AND THEIR ANSWERS

VOTE OF THANKS

FOREWARD

Welcome to Breaking Free from Asthma! Your Essential Guide to Managing and Overcoming Respiratory Challenges. Whether you or someone you care about is coping with asthma, you know firsthand the daily impact it can have—managing symptoms, navigating treatments, and understanding triggers. This comprehensive guide is crafted to empower you with knowledge and practical strategies for taking charge of your respiratory health.

Within these pages, we will explore the essentials of asthma, effective management techniques, and key topics such as forming a supportive healthcare team, identifying asthma triggers, and optimizing medication usage. Whether you're newly diagnosed or have been living with asthma for years, this book aims to offer valuable insights and resources to help you live well and thrive despite the challenges posed by this chronic condition.

Remember, you are not alone on this journey. Armed with the right information and proactive management, you can overcome the constraints of asthma and lead a fulfilling life. Let's embark together on this empowering path towards improved respiratory health and a brighter future.

CHAPTER 1: UNDERSTANDING THE FUNDAMENTALS OF ASTHMA

Asthma is a chronic respiratory condition that impacts millions worldwide, posing significant challenges to breathing and overall well-being. From childhood to adulthood, grasping the essentials of asthma is pivotal for effective management and enhancing daily life quality.

What is Asthma?

Asthma involves inflammation and narrowing of the airways, leading to breathing difficulties. This condition manifests through recurring episodes of wheezing, breathlessness, chest tightness, and coughing, often exacerbated at night or in the early morning. Symptoms vary in intensity among individuals, ranging from mild discomfort to severe respiratory distress.

The core issue in asthma lies in the airway inflammation triggered by allergens (like pollen, dust mites, and pet dander), respiratory infections, physical exertion, cold air, smoke, and certain chemicals. This inflammation prompts excessive mucus production, further constricting the air passages and hindering normal airflow into and out of the lungs.

Common Symptoms of Asthma

Recognizing asthma symptoms is critical for prompt intervention and effective management. Key symptoms include:

- **Wheezing:** Audible whistling or squeaking sounds during breathing, especially during exhalation.
- **Shortness Of Breath:** Difficulty in breathing, feeling unable to fully catch one's breath.

- **Chest Tightness:** Sensation of pressure or constriction in the chest.
- **Coughing:** Often worsened at night or early morning, exacerbated by cold air or physical exertion.

Symptoms may vary in frequency and severity. Some individuals experience occasional mild symptoms, while others contend with severe asthma that significantly impacts daily activities, necessitating ongoing management.

Types of Asthma

Asthma presents in various forms, each influenced by distinct triggers and patterns:

- **Allergic Asthma:** Triggered by exposure to allergens such as pollen, dust mites, mold, or animal dander, prompting asthma symptoms in susceptible individuals.

- **Non-Allergic Asthma:** Triggered by factors other than allergens, including respiratory infections (e.g., colds, flu), physical activity, cold air, smoke, or strong odors.

- **Occupational Asthma:** Develops due to exposure to workplace irritants such as chemicals, gases, dust, or fumes, affecting individuals in diverse professions, from industrial workers to healthcare providers.

- **Childhood Asthma:** Often associated with allergies, frequently improving with age. Early diagnosis and management are crucial to reducing symptoms and optimizing lung function development.

Causes and Risk Factors

While the precise cause of asthma remains unclear, several factors contribute to its onset and exacerbation:

- **Genetic Predisposition:** Asthma tends to run in families, indicating a genetic predisposition. Individuals with a family history of asthma or allergies are at higher risk.

- **Environmental Factors:** Exposure to allergens, air pollution, tobacco smoke, and early-life respiratory infections heightens the likelihood of developing asthma.

- **Early Childhood Exposures:** Infants exposed to allergens or respiratory infections are more prone to developing asthma later in life.

Understanding these risk factors helps individuals and healthcare providers identify potential triggers and implement preventive measures for effective asthma management.

Diagnosis of Asthma

Diagnosing asthma involves a thorough evaluation by a healthcare professional, encompassing:

- **Medical History:** Gathering information on symptoms, family history of asthma or allergies, and environmental exposures.

- **Physical Examination:** Assessing lung function, listening for abnormal chest sounds like wheezing, and evaluating overall respiratory health.

- **Lung Function Tests:** Conducting spirometry to measure lung capacity and peak flow tests to monitor airflow in the lungs.

- **Allergy Testing:** Identifying specific allergens that may trigger asthma symptoms through skin or blood tests (allergen-specific IgE testing).

A comprehensive diagnostic approach distinguishes asthma from other respiratory conditions and guides the formulation of a personalized treatment plan.

Treatment Approaches

Managing asthma entails a multifaceted approach tailored to individual needs:

- **Medications:** Using bronchodilators (e.g., short-acting beta-agonists) to alleviate acute symptoms and anti-inflammatory drugs (e.g., corticosteroids) to reduce airway inflammation and prevent asthma attacks.

- **Allergen Avoidance:** Identifying and minimizing exposure to allergens such as dust mites, pollen, mold, and animal dander.

- **Asthma Action Plan:** Collaborating with healthcare providers to create a personalized plan outlining daily management strategies, recognizing symptom exacerbations, and knowing when to seek medical help.

- Lifestyle Modifications: Embracing healthy habits like regular physical activity (with appropriate precautions), maintaining a smoke-free environment, and effectively managing stress.

Conclusion

Comprehending the fundamentals of asthma is pivotal for individuals managing this chronic respiratory condition. By recognizing symptoms, identifying triggers, and partnering closely with healthcare providers, individuals can effectively manage asthma and enhance their quality of life. This chapter has offered an overview of asthma's definition, symptoms, types, causes, diagnosis, and treatment strategies. In subsequent chapters, we will delve deeper into strategies for building a supportive healthcare team, optimizing medication use, and thriving with asthma. Together, let's empower ourselves to overcome the challenges of asthma and embrace a healthier, more active lifestyle.

CHAPTER 2: BUILDING YOUR HEALTHCARE SUPPORT TEAM

Effective management of asthma relies heavily on establishing a supportive healthcare team that comprehends your specific needs and collaborates to enhance your respiratory well-being. This chapter delves into the essential elements of your healthcare support team, from primary care providers to specialists, and provides guidance on creating and maintaining a proactive partnership for effective asthma management.

The Role of Your Primary Care Provider

Your primary care provider (PCP) acts as the cornerstone of your healthcare team. Typically your family doctor or general practitioner, they oversee your overall health and coordinate your asthma care. Their responsibilities in asthma management include:

- **Diagnosis and Initial Treatment:** Your PCP often makes the initial diagnosis of asthma based on symptoms, medical history, and diagnostic tests. They may start treatment with medications and provide initial education on managing asthma.

- **Regular Monitoring:** Your PCP monitors your asthma symptoms, lung function, and overall health during routine check-ups. They assess the effectiveness of treatments and make adjustments when necessary.

- **Referrals to Specialists:** If your asthma requires specialized care due to complexity or difficulty in control, your PCP may refer you to specialists such as allergists, pulmonologists, or respiratory therapists for further evaluation and focused care.

The Role of Specialists in Asthma Care

Depending on the severity of your asthma and your specific needs, your healthcare team may include various specialists who play crucial roles in managing and optimizing your respiratory health:

- **Allergists/Immunologists:** Experts in diagnosing and treating allergies and allergic asthma. They conduct allergy tests to identify specific triggers and develop personalized treatment plans that may include allergen immunotherapy.

- **Pulmonologists:** Specialize in respiratory diseases, including asthma.

They assess lung function, perform advanced diagnostic tests (like spirometry and bronchial provocation tests), and manage severe or complex cases of asthma.

- Respiratory Therapists: Trained in assessing lung function and administering breathing treatments. They educate patients on proper inhaler techniques, monitor asthma symptoms, and provide guidance on using respiratory devices effectively.

- Pediatricians or Pediatric Pulmonologists: Specialize in treating children with asthma. They customize asthma management plans to suit children's unique developmental needs and offer guidance to parents on managing asthma in young children.

Other Members of Your Healthcare Team

Beyond primary care providers and specialists, several other healthcare professionals contribute to comprehensive asthma care:

- **Nurses:** Assist in asthma education, symptom monitoring, and treatment administration in clinical settings. They also offer ongoing support and guidance for managing asthma at home.

- **Pharmacists:** Provide expertise on medications used to treat asthma, including inhalers, corticosteroids, and bronchodilators. They ensure patients understand how to use their medications correctly and may offer counseling on managing asthma symptoms.

- **Nutritionists/Dietitians:** Offer guidance on nutrition and dietary habits that support respiratory health. They may suggest dietary changes to manage inflammation or address nutritional deficiencies affecting asthma control.

Establishing Effective Communication

Effective communication is crucial for fostering a collaborative relationship with your healthcare team. Consider these strategies to improve communication and maximize the benefits of your asthma care:

- **Prepare for Appointments:** Before each visit, note down any symptoms or concerns since your last appointment. Bring a list of current medications and be ready to discuss any changes in your asthma symptoms.

- **Ask Questions:** Don't hesitate to ask your healthcare providers about your asthma management plan, treatment options, potential medication side effects, and strategies for improving asthma control.

- **Share Updates:** Keep your healthcare team informed about changes in your asthma symptoms, triggers you've identified, or challenges you're facing in managing your condition. Open communication enables them to adjust your treatment plan accordingly.

- **Follow Up:** Schedule regular follow-up appointments as advised by your healthcare providers. These visits allow for ongoing assessment of asthma control, adjustment of medications, and evaluation of any new symptoms or concerns.

Collaborating for Personalized Care

Each member of your healthcare team brings unique expertise to your asthma care. By collaborating effectively and actively participating in your treatment plan, you can optimize asthma management and enhance your quality of life. Remember, your healthcare team is dedicated to supporting you in overcoming the challenges of asthma and achieving better respiratory health.

Conclusion

Establishing a robust healthcare support team is fundamental to effectively managing asthma and overcoming respiratory challenges. Your primary care provider, specialists, and other healthcare professionals collaborate to diagnose asthma, tailor treatment plans, monitor your condition, and provide ongoing support and education. By fostering open communication, asking questions, and actively engaging in your asthma care, you empower yourself to take charge of your respiratory health and enjoy life to the fullest. In upcoming chapters, we will explore strategies for optimizing medication usage, identifying and managing asthma triggers, and thriving with asthma across various stages of life. Together, let's continue on the journey to breaking free from asthma and embracing a healthier future.

CHAPTER 3: MAXIMIZING YOUR DOCTOR VISITS

Effectively managing asthma requires a strong partnership between you and your healthcare provider. Making sure each visit to your doctor is as productive as possible is crucial for gaining control over your asthma and improving your overall quality of life. This chapter provides guidance on how to prepare for appointments, understand your treatment plan, and communicate effectively with your doctor to maximize each visit.

Preparing for Your Appointment

Proper preparation is essential to make the most of your doctor's visit. Here's how to get ready:

1. Maintain a Symptom Diary: Record your symptoms, noting their frequency, severity, and any triggers. Include information about nighttime awakenings, limitations on physical activities, and how often you use your rescue inhaler. This data helps your doctor evaluate the severity of your asthma and the effectiveness of your current treatment.

2. Compile a Medication List: Write down all the medications you take, including dosages and frequency. Don't forget to include over-the-counter drugs, supplements, and herbal remedies. Bring this list to your appointment so your doctor can review your current regimen.

3. Prepare Questions and Concerns: Think about any questions or concerns you have about your asthma. Write them down and bring the list with you to ensure you don't forget to address important issues during your visit.

4. Review Your Action Plan: If you have an asthma action plan, review it and note any difficulties or areas needing clarification. If you don't have one, discuss creating a plan with your doctor during your visit.

During the Appointment

Effective communication with your doctor is crucial. Here are some tips to help you get the most out of your appointment:

1. Be Honest and Transparent: Share all relevant information about your symptoms, lifestyle, and how you manage your asthma. Being honest is vital for accurate assessments and recommendations.

2. Clearly Describe Symptoms: Provide specific details when describing your symptoms. Instead of saying, "I feel short of breath," explain when it happens, what activities trigger it, and how long it lasts. This helps your doctor better understand your condition.

3. Discuss Triggers and Lifestyle Factors: Talk about known triggers like allergens, exercise, stress, or environmental factors. Discuss lifestyle changes or new stressors that might be affecting your asthma. Your doctor can offer advice on managing these triggers.

4. Inquire About Medication Side Effects: If you experience side effects from medications, inform your doctor. They can adjust your treatment plan or suggest alternatives to minimize these effects.

5. Understand Your Treatment Plan: Make sure you fully understand your treatment plan, including how and when to take your medications. Ask your doctor to clarify anything that is unclear. Following your treatment plan precisely is essential for effective asthma management.

6. Review Your Asthma Action Plan: Go over your asthma action plan with your doctor to ensure it's up-to-date and that you understand each step. Your plan should include instructions on handling worsening symptoms, using your rescue inhaler, and when to seek emergency care.

After the Appointment

Following up after your appointment is as important as preparing for and attending the visit. Here's what to do:

1. Implement Doctor's Recommendations: Start any new medications or treatments as prescribed. Make suggested lifestyle changes and monitor their effects on your asthma.

2. Update Your Symptom Diary: Continue tracking your symptoms and any changes due to your new treatment plan. This information will be valuable for your next appointment.

3. Maintain Communication: If you have questions or concerns after your appointment, contact your doctor. Prompt communication can help address issues before they become more significant problems.

4. Schedule Follow-Up Appointments: Regular follow-up visits are essential for monitoring your asthma and making necessary treatment adjustments. Ensure you schedule and attend these appointments.

Utilizing Your Healthcare Team

Besides your primary care doctor or pulmonologist, other healthcare professionals can help manage your asthma:

1. Allergists: If allergies significantly trigger your asthma, an allergist can identify specific allergens and recommend treatments, like allergy shots, to reduce sensitivity.

2. Respiratory Therapists: They provide education on proper inhaler techniques, breathing exercises, and strategies to improve lung function and control asthma.

3. Pharmacists: Pharmacists offer valuable information about medications, including potential interactions, proper usage, and managing side effects. They can also help you understand how to use devices like inhalers and nebulizers correctly.

4. Dietitians: A dietitian can help create a balanced diet that supports overall health and reduces inflammation, beneficial for managing asthma.

5. Physical Therapists: If physical activity triggers your asthma, a physical therapist can develop an exercise plan to help you stay active while minimizing asthma symptoms.

Advocating for Yourself

Being an active participant in your healthcare is crucial for managing asthma effectively. Here's how to advocate for yourself:

1. Educate Yourself: Learn about asthma, its triggers, and treatments. The more you know, the better equipped you'll be to manage your condition and communicate with your healthcare team.

2. Speak Up: If your concerns aren't being addressed or you have questions about your treatment plan, speak up. Your input is valuable to your healthcare team.

3. Seek Second Opinions: If you're not satisfied with your current treatment or if your asthma isn't well-controlled, seek a second opinion. A different perspective can provide new insights and options.

4. Join Support Groups: Connecting with others who have asthma can provide emotional support and practical advice. Support groups are also valuable for learning about new treatments and strategies for managing asthma.

Conclusion

Maximizing your doctor visits is essential for managing asthma effectively. By preparing thoroughly, communicating clearly, and following up diligently, you can ensure each appointment moves you closer to better asthma control. Remember, managing asthma is a collaborative effort between you and your healthcare team. With the right approach, you can take charge of your asthma and lead a healthy, active life.

CHAPTER 4: Achieving Wellness with Asthma

Living with asthma presents its challenges, but it doesn't prevent you from achieving overall wellness. Wellness is a holistic concept that includes managing asthma effectively while also tending to your physical, emotional, and mental health. This chapter explores various strategies to help you maintain a balanced and healthy lifestyle while managing asthma.

Understanding Wellness

Wellness extends beyond the absence of illness; it involves thriving in all areas of life. For those with asthma, achieving wellness means managing the condition effectively to minimize its impact on daily life. This comprehensive approach includes lifestyle changes, stress management, proper medication use, physical activity, and mental health care.

Developing a Healthy Lifestyle

Maintaining a healthy lifestyle is crucial for managing asthma and promoting overall wellness. Key components include:

1. Balanced Diet: Nutrition significantly impacts overall health and asthma control. A diet rich in fruits, vegetables, whole grains, and lean proteins can reduce inflammation and boost the immune system. Avoiding food triggers, such as sulfites in processed foods, can help prevent asthma flare-ups.

2. Regular Exercise: Physical activity is important for cardiovascular health and overall fitness, but asthma can make exercise challenging. Work with your doctor to create an exercise plan that suits your needs. Activities like swimming, walking, or yoga can be beneficial as they are less likely to trigger asthma symptoms. Always warm up before exercising and keep your rescue inhaler nearby.

3. Adequate Sleep: Quality sleep is essential for both physical and mental health. Asthma can sometimes disrupt sleep, particularly if symptoms worsen at night. Maintaining good sleep hygiene, such as a regular sleep schedule and a comfortable sleep environment, can improve sleep quality. If asthma symptoms interfere with sleep, consult your doctor about adjusting your treatment plan.

4. Avoiding Triggers: Identifying and avoiding asthma triggers is crucial for managing the condition. Common triggers include allergens (like pollen, dust mites, and pet dander), smoke, air pollution, cold air, and respiratory infections. Using air purifiers, keeping your home clean, and avoiding smoke and other irritants can help minimize triggers.

Managing Stress

Stress can worsen asthma symptoms, making effective stress management vital for achieving wellness. Strategies to manage stress include:

1. Mindfulness and Meditation: Mindfulness practices and meditation can help reduce stress and promote relaxation. These techniques encourage focusing on the present moment and can be particularly helpful in managing asthma-related anxiety.

2. Breathing Exercises: Breathing exercises can improve lung function and reduce stress. Techniques like diaphragmatic breathing, pursed-lip breathing, and the Buteyko method can help manage asthma symptoms and promote relaxation.

3. Physical Activity: Regular exercise benefits physical health, reduces stress, and improves mood. Engaging in enjoyable activities like walking, swimming, or yoga can provide both physical and mental health benefits.

4. Support Systems: Having a strong support system is important for managing stress. Connecting with friends, family, support groups, or a mental health professional can provide emotional support and practical advice for managing asthma.

Medication Management

Proper medication management is essential for controlling asthma and maintaining wellness. Tips for effective management include:

1. Adherence to Treatment: Follow your prescribed treatment plan, taking medications as directed. Adhering to your medication regimen helps prevent asthma attacks and keeps symptoms under control.

2. Regular Check-Ups: Regular visits to your healthcare provider are essential for monitoring asthma control and making necessary adjustments to your treatment plan. Use these visits to discuss any concerns or changes in your symptoms.

3. Understanding Medications: Understand the purpose and proper use of each medication you take. Know the difference between long-term control medications, which prevent symptoms, and rescue medications, which provide quick relief during an asthma attack.

4. Asthma Action Plan: Work with your doctor to develop and maintain an asthma action plan. This plan outlines how to manage daily asthma symptoms and handle worsening symptoms or asthma attacks. Ensure you understand and follow the plan.

Mental Health Care

Mental health is an important aspect of overall wellness, especially for those with chronic conditions like asthma. Ways to care for your mental health include:

1. Therapy and Counseling: Therapy or counseling can help manage the emotional challenges of living with asthma. Cognitive-behavioral therapy (CBT) can be particularly effective in addressing anxiety and depression.

2. Stress-Relief Activities: Engage in activities that bring joy and relaxation, such as hobbies, spending time with loved ones, or practicing mindfulness. These activities can help reduce stress and improve your mood.

3. Education and Empowerment: Educate yourself about asthma to feel more in control of your condition. Understanding asthma and how to manage it can reduce anxiety and empower you to take an active role in your health.

Integrative and Complementary Approaches

Some people find relief and improved wellness through integrative and complementary approaches. Always discuss these with your doctor before trying them:

1. Acupuncture: Some studies suggest acupuncture may help reduce asthma symptoms by improving airflow and reducing inflammation.

2. Herbal Remedies: Certain herbs and supplements, such as ginger, turmeric, and omega-3 fatty acids, may have anti-inflammatory properties that benefit asthma. However, always consult your doctor before starting any new supplements.

3. Aromatherapy: Using essential oils like eucalyptus or lavender can promote relaxation and potentially improve breathing. Be cautious, as some scents can trigger asthma symptoms in sensitive individuals.

Conclusion

Achieving wellness with asthma involves a holistic approach that includes managing your condition effectively while taking care of your physical, emotional, and mental health. By adopting a healthy lifestyle, managing stress, adhering to your treatment plan, and caring for your mental health, you can live a fulfilling and active life with asthma. Wellness is an ongoing journey that requires continuous effort and commitment, but with the right strategies and support, you can break free from the limitations of asthma and thrive.

CHAPTER 5: LONG-TERM ASTHMA MANAGEMENT

Managing asthma effectively over the long term requires a strategic and consistent approach. This involves not just managing daily symptoms but also preventing severe asthma attacks and maintaining overall health. Long-term asthma management includes creating a detailed plan, continuous monitoring, lifestyle modifications, and staying well-informed about the condition. This chapter offers comprehensive strategies for effective long-term asthma management.

Understanding Long-Term Asthma Management

Asthma is a chronic disease that inflames and narrows the airways. Effective long-term management focuses on keeping asthma under control by reducing inflammation, preventing exacerbations, and maintaining optimal lung function. This is achieved through a combination of medications, lifestyle changes, and regular medical supervision.

Developing a Comprehensive Asthma Management Plan

An effective asthma management plan is crucial for long-term control. This plan should be tailored to your specific needs and developed in consultation with your healthcare provider. Key elements of a robust asthma management plan include:

1. Medication Plan: Understand your prescribed medications, including long-term control drugs (like inhaled corticosteroids) and quick-relief medications (like bronchodilators). Follow your doctor's instructions on how and when to use these medications.

2. Asthma Action Plan: Collaborate with your healthcare provider to create an asthma action plan. This plan should outline daily management techniques, recognize signs of worsening asthma, and provide clear steps for handling asthma attacks. Keep this plan accessible and share it with family members and caregivers.

3. Regular Monitoring: Track your asthma regularly to see how well your management plan is working. This could involve keeping a symptom diary, using a peak flow meter to measure lung function, and noting any triggers or patterns in your symptoms.

Medication Adherence and Management

Consistently taking your medications as prescribed is essential for long-term asthma control. Here are some tips for effective medication management:

1. Adherence to Medication: Take your long-term control medications regularly, even when you feel fine. These medications help prevent symptoms and reduce airway inflammation. Missing doses can lead to loss of asthma control.

2. Understanding Your Medications: Know the purpose of each medication and how to use it correctly. Long-term control medications prevent symptoms, while quick-relief medications provide immediate relief during asthma attacks. Using a spacer with your inhaler can improve medication delivery to the lungs.

3. Regular Medical Reviews: Have regular check-ups with your healthcare provider to review your asthma management plan. Discuss any changes in symptoms, medication side effects, and any concerns you have. Your doctor may adjust your treatment plan based on your current condition.

Identifying and Avoiding Triggers

Identifying and avoiding asthma triggers is a key part of long-term management. Common triggers include allergens, respiratory infections, exercise, cold air, smoke, and stress. Strategies to minimize exposure to triggers include:

1. Allergen Control: Reduce exposure to indoor allergens like dust mites, pet dander, mold, and pollen. Use allergen-proof mattress and pillow covers, regularly clean and vacuum your home, and keep windows closed during high pollen seasons.

2. Avoiding Smoke and Pollution: Avoid exposure to tobacco smoke, secondhand smoke, and air pollution. Stay indoors on days with poor air quality and use air purifiers to reduce indoor air pollutants.

3. Infection Prevention: Respiratory infections can worsen asthma symptoms. Practice good hygiene, get vaccinated against the flu and pneumonia, and avoid close contact with people who have respiratory infections.

4. Exercise Management: Physical activity is important for overall health but can sometimes trigger asthma symptoms. Choose activities less likely to cause symptoms, like swimming, walking, or cycling. Warm up before exercising and use your quick-relief inhaler if needed before physical activity.

Lifestyle Adjustments for Long-Term Control

Making lifestyle changes can help manage asthma more effectively. Consider the following strategies:

1. Healthy Diet: A balanced diet rich in fruits, vegetables, whole grains, and lean proteins supports overall health and reduces inflammation. Some studies suggest omega-3 fatty acids found in fish oil may help improve asthma symptoms.

2. Regular Exercise: Regular physical activity improves lung function, reduces stress, and enhances overall well-being. Choose activities you enjoy that are suitable for your asthma condition. Always carry your quick-relief inhaler when exercising.

3. Stress Management: Stress can trigger or worsen asthma symptoms. Practice stress-reducing techniques like mindfulness, meditation, deep breathing exercises, and yoga. Ensure you have a support system to help manage stress effectively.

4. Adequate Sleep: Quality sleep is essential for maintaining good health and managing asthma. Establish a regular sleep routine, create a comfortable sleep environment, and address any factors that may disrupt your sleep, such as nighttime asthma symptoms.

Staying Informed and Empowered

Staying informed about asthma and its management is crucial for long-term control. Consider these tips:

1. Education: Learn about asthma, its triggers, and the latest treatments. Understanding your condition helps you take an active role in managing it and making informed decisions about your health.

2. Support Groups: Join asthma support groups or online communities to connect with others who have asthma. Sharing experiences and tips provides valuable insights and emotional support.

3. Communication with Healthcare Providers: Maintain open communication with your healthcare team. Don't hesitate to ask questions, seek clarification, or discuss any concerns you have about your asthma management.

Conclusion

Effective long-term asthma management requires a comprehensive and proactive approach. By developing a personalized asthma management plan, adhering to medication regimens, identifying and avoiding triggers, making lifestyle adjustments, and staying informed, you can effectively control your asthma and lead a healthy, active life. Remember, managing asthma is an ongoing process, but with the right strategies and support, you can break free from asthma's limitations and achieve long-term wellness.

CHAPTER 6: IDENTIFYING ASTHMA TRIGGERS

Asthma is a chronic respiratory condition significantly influenced by various environmental and internal factors, known as triggers. Recognizing and managing these triggers is crucial for controlling asthma symptoms and preventing flare-ups. This chapter explores different types of asthma triggers, methods to identify them, and strategies to effectively avoid or manage them.

Understanding Asthma Triggers

Asthma triggers are substances or conditions that can cause the airways to become inflamed and narrow, leading to symptoms like coughing, wheezing, shortness of breath, and chest tightness. Triggers vary widely among individuals, making it essential to understand your specific triggers for effective asthma management. Triggers can be broadly categorized into allergenic and non-allergenic types.

Allergenic Triggers

Allergenic triggers cause allergic reactions, which can trigger asthma symptoms. Common allergenic triggers include:

1. Pollen: Pollen from trees, grasses, and weeds is a common trigger, particularly during certain seasons. Monitoring pollen counts and staying indoors on high-pollen days can help reduce exposure.

2. Dust Mites: These microscopic creatures thrive in household dust, bedding, and upholstered furniture. Using allergen-proof covers on mattresses and pillows, washing bedding in hot water, and keeping a clean home can reduce dust mite exposure.

3. Pet Dander: Proteins found in the skin flakes, urine, and saliva of pets can trigger asthma symptoms. Keeping pets out of bedrooms, regularly bathing and grooming pets, and using air purifiers can help manage this trigger.

4. Mold: Mold spores in damp areas such as bathrooms, kitchens, and basements can be significant triggers. Reducing indoor humidity, fixing leaks, and cleaning moldy surfaces with appropriate cleaners can control mold growth.

5. Cockroaches: The droppings, saliva, and body parts of cockroaches can trigger asthma. Keeping your home clean, sealing cracks and crevices, and using bait or traps can help manage cockroach infestations.

Non-Allergenic Triggers

Non-allergenic triggers can also cause asthma symptoms and are often related to environmental factors, lifestyle choices, or health conditions. Common non-allergenic triggers include:

1. Respiratory Infections: Infections such as the common cold, flu, or sinusitis can worsen asthma symptoms. Practicing good hygiene, getting vaccinated, and managing infections promptly can help mitigate this trigger.

2. Exercise: Physical activity, especially in cold or dry air, can trigger asthma symptoms in some individuals. Warming up before exercise, using quick-relief inhalers before physical activity, and choosing appropriate exercises can help manage exercise-induced asthma.

3. Cold Air: Breathing in cold, dry air can irritate the airways and trigger asthma symptoms. Wearing a scarf or mask over the nose and mouth in cold weather can help warm and humidify the air before it enters the lungs.

4. Air Pollutants: Exposure to outdoor pollutants such as smog, car exhaust, and industrial emissions can worsen asthma. Staying indoors on days with poor air quality and using air purifiers can help reduce exposure.

5. Tobacco Smoke: Smoking and exposure to secondhand smoke are significant asthma triggers. Quitting smoking and avoiding environments where smoking occurs can greatly improve asthma control.

6. Strong Odors and Chemicals: Perfumes, cleaning products, and other strong odors can irritate the airways. Using fragrance-free products and ensuring proper ventilation when using chemicals can help avoid this trigger.

Identifying Your Asthma Triggers

Identifying your specific asthma triggers is vital for managing your condition. Here are some strategies to help you identify your triggers:

1. Keep a Symptom Diary: Record your symptoms, their severity, and any potential triggers you encountered each day. Over time, patterns may emerge that can help you pinpoint specific triggers.

2. Use a Peak Flow Meter: Regularly monitoring your lung function with a peak flow meter can help identify triggers. A decrease in peak flow readings may indicate exposure to a trigger.

3. Allergy Testing: Consult your healthcare provider about allergy testing. Skin prick tests or blood tests can identify specific allergens that may be triggering your asthma.

4. Environmental Assessments: Evaluate your home and work environments for potential triggers. This can include checking for mold, dust, and other allergens, as well as assessing air quality.

Managing and Avoiding Triggers

Once you have identified your asthma triggers, taking steps to manage and avoid them is crucial. Here are some effective strategies:

1. Create an Allergen-Free Environment: Implement measures to reduce exposure to indoor allergens. Use air purifiers, maintain low humidity levels, and clean regularly to minimize dust and mold.

2. Practice Good Hygiene: Regular handwashing, avoiding close contact with sick individuals, and getting vaccinated can help prevent respiratory infections that trigger asthma.

3. Exercise Smart: Choose activities that are less likely to trigger symptoms, such as swimming or walking. Warm up before exercise and use a quick-relief inhaler if recommended by your healthcare provider.

4. Monitor Air Quality: Stay informed about local air quality levels and limit outdoor activities on days with high pollution. Use air purifiers at home to maintain clean indoor air.

5. Quit Smoking: If you smoke, seek support to quit. Avoid exposure to secondhand smoke and environments where smoking is prevalent.

6. Manage Stress: Stress can exacerbate asthma symptoms. Practice stress-relief techniques such as mindfulness, meditation, and yoga to maintain emotional well-being.
\

Conclusion

Identifying and managing asthma triggers is an ongoing process that requires vigilance and proactive measures. By understanding the various triggers and how they affect your asthma, you can take steps to avoid or minimize exposure, leading to better control over your symptoms and a higher quality of life. Remember, working closely with your healthcare provider to develop a personalized asthma management plan is essential for long-term success. With the right strategies in place, you can break free from the limitations of asthma and enjoy a healthier, more active life.

CHAPTER 7: INHALANT ALLERGIES AND THEIR IMPACT

Inhalant allergies are a significant concern for people with asthma as they can worsen symptoms and lead to severe respiratory problems. Understanding the link between inhalant allergies and asthma, and learning how to manage these allergies, is essential for maintaining good respiratory health and overall well-being. This chapter delves into the various types of inhalant allergies, their impact on asthma, and effective strategies to manage and reduce their effects.

What are Inhalant Allergies?

Inhalant allergies occur when the immune system reacts to airborne substances like pollen, dust mites, pet dander, mold spores, and other environmental allergens. For asthmatics, exposure to these allergens can lead to airway inflammation and hyperresponsiveness, causing asthma symptoms such as wheezing, coughing, shortness of breath, and chest tightness. Identifying and managing these allergens is crucial in controlling asthma.

Common Inhalant Allergens

Inhalant allergens can be divided into seasonal and perennial categories. Seasonal allergens appear at specific times of the year, while perennial allergens are present year-round.

1. Pollen: One of the most common inhalant allergens, pollen from trees, grasses, and weeds can trigger allergic reactions and asthma symptoms. Pollen allergies often vary with the season, with spring and fall being particularly challenging.

2. Dust Mites: These microscopic organisms live in household dust, bedding, and upholstered furniture.

Dust mite allergies can cause persistent asthma symptoms due to constant exposure in the home.

3. Pet Dander: Proteins found in the skin flakes, urine, and saliva of pets can trigger asthma symptoms. Even indirect contact with pets can be problematic, as dander can spread through the air and settle on surfaces.

4. Mold Spores: Mold grows in damp, humid environments and releases spores into the air, which can trigger asthma symptoms. Common areas where mold can be found include bathrooms, basements, and kitchens.

5. Cockroach Droppings: Cockroach allergens can become airborne and trigger asthma symptoms. These allergens are often found in homes, especially in urban areas.

Impact of Inhalant Allergies on Asthma

The relationship between inhalant allergies and asthma is complex. Inhalant allergens can worsen asthma symptoms through various mechanisms:

1. Airway Inflammation: Inhalant allergens can cause airway inflammation, leading to swelling and increased mucus production, making breathing more difficult and triggering asthma symptoms.

2. Hyperresponsiveness: Exposure to inhalant allergens can make the airways more sensitive to other triggers, such as cold air, exercise, and respiratory infections, resulting in more frequent and severe asthma attacks.

3. Immune System Activation: Inhalant allergens can activate the immune system, leading to the release of inflammatory mediators like histamines, which contribute to asthma symptoms.

4. Chronic Exposure: Continuous exposure to inhalant allergens can lead to chronic inflammation and airway remodeling, changing the structure of the airways over time. This can result in long-term respiratory issues and decreased lung function.

Managing Inhalant Allergies

Managing inhalant allergies effectively is crucial for controlling asthma symptoms and improving quality of life. Here are some strategies to help manage inhalant allergies:

1. Identify Allergens: Work with your healthcare provider to identify specific inhalant allergens that trigger your asthma symptoms. This can be done through allergy testing, such as skin prick tests or blood tests.

2. Reduce Exposure: Once you know your triggers, take steps to reduce exposure to these allergens. This may involve changes in your home environment, such as using allergen-proof covers on mattresses and pillows, removing carpets, and regularly cleaning to reduce dust and pet dander.

3. Monitor Pollen Counts: During high-pollen seasons, stay indoors as much as possible, especially on windy days. Keep windows closed and use air conditioning to filter the air. Shower and change clothes after spending time outdoors to remove pollen.

4. Control Humidity: Reduce indoor humidity levels to prevent mold growth. Use dehumidifiers, fix leaks promptly, and ensure good ventilation in damp areas like bathrooms and kitchens.

5. Use Air Purifiers: High-efficiency particulate air (HEPA) filters can help remove airborne allergens from your home. Consider using HEPA filters in your bedroom and other frequently used areas.

6. Regular Cleaning: Clean your home regularly to reduce the buildup of dust, pet dander, and other allergens. Use a vacuum cleaner with a HEPA filter and wash bedding in hot water weekly.

7. Pet Management: If you have pets, keep them out of bedrooms and off furniture. Bathe and groom them regularly to reduce dander. Consider using air purifiers to help manage pet allergens.

8. Medications: Your healthcare provider may recommend medications to manage your allergies and asthma. These may include antihistamines, nasal corticosteroids, and leukotriene modifiers. Quick-relief inhalers and long-term asthma control medications can also help manage symptoms.

9. Immunotherapy: For severe allergies, immunotherapy (allergy shots or sublingual tablets) may be an option. This treatment involves gradually exposing the body to small amounts of the allergen to build up tolerance and reduce symptoms over time.

Conclusion

Inhalant allergies play a significant role in triggering and worsening asthma symptoms. Understanding the connection between these allergens and asthma is crucial for effective management. By identifying specific inhalant allergens and implementing strategies to reduce exposure, individuals with asthma can significantly improve their respiratory health and quality of life. Remember to work closely with your healthcare provider to develop a personalized asthma and allergy management plan that addresses your unique needs and triggers. With the right approach, you can break free from the limitations imposed by inhalant allergies and asthma, leading to a healthier, more active life.

CHAPTER 8: FOOD ALLERGIES AND ASTHMA

Food allergies can have a profound impact on individuals with asthma, worsening symptoms and complicating treatment. Understanding how food allergies interact with asthma, identifying common triggers, and implementing effective management strategies are crucial for maintaining optimal respiratory health. This chapter delves into the intersection of food allergies and asthma, offering insights into their effects and practical advice for managing both conditions.

The Connection Between Food Allergies and Asthma

Food allergies occur when the immune system reacts to proteins in certain foods, triggering allergic responses that can affect the respiratory system in people with asthma. Consuming allergenic foods can lead to asthma symptoms such as wheezing, coughing, and shortness of breath, ranging from mild discomfort to severe, life-threatening anaphylaxis. For individuals with asthma, awareness of potential food allergens is essential to prevent exacerbations.

Common Food Allergens

Several foods are known to trigger allergic reactions in individuals with asthma and other allergies. These include:

1. Peanuts: Peanut allergies can cause severe reactions, including anaphylaxis. Peanut allergens are widespread and can be found in processed foods and restaurant dishes, posing challenges for complete avoidance.

2. Tree Nuts: Allergies to tree nuts like almonds, walnuts, and cashews can also provoke allergic reactions in asthmatics. Cross-contamination in food manufacturing is a significant concern.

3. Shellfish: Shellfish allergies are common and can result in serious allergic reactions in sensitive individuals. Those with shellfish allergies should exercise caution when dining out or consuming processed foods.

4. Milk: Milk allergies involve reactions to proteins in cow's milk and can trigger respiratory symptoms in individuals with asthma. Dairy products are ubiquitous in diets, making avoidance difficult.

5. Eggs: Egg allergies can affect both children and adults, causing respiratory distress in asthmatics. Eggs are prevalent in baked goods and processed foods, increasing the risk of accidental exposure.

6. Wheat: Wheat allergies involve immune responses to proteins in wheat products. Asthmatics with wheat allergies may experience respiratory symptoms if exposed to wheat-containing foods.

7. Soy: Soy allergies can provoke allergic reactions in individuals with asthma. Soy is used in various processed foods, making complete avoidance challenging.

Impact of Food Allergies on Asthma

Food allergies can significantly exacerbate asthma symptoms through various mechanisms:

1. Immediate Reactions: Consuming allergenic foods can trigger immediate allergic reactions, leading to respiratory distress in individuals with asthma.

2. Systemic Inflammation: Food allergies can cause systemic inflammation, aggravating airway inflammation in asthmatics and making breathing more challenging.

3. Anaphylaxis: Severe food allergies can induce anaphylactic reactions, characterized by sudden and severe respiratory symptoms like airway constriction and difficulty breathing.

4. Delayed Reactions: Some food allergies can result in delayed allergic responses, complicating the identification of specific allergens triggering asthma symptoms.

Managing Food Allergies and Asthma

Effective management of food allergies and asthma involves several strategies to minimize allergic reactions and maintain respiratory health:

1. Identify Allergic Triggers: Collaborate with allergists or healthcare providers to identify specific food allergens that trigger asthma symptoms. Allergy tests such as skin prick tests or blood tests can pinpoint allergenic foods.

2. Avoid Exposure: Once allergens are identified, take precautions to avoid exposure. Read food labels meticulously, inquire about ingredients when dining out, and remain vigilant about cross-contamination during food preparation.

3. Create a Safe Environment: Ensure that home environments are free from allergenic foods. Use separate utensils and cooking equipment for allergen-free meals, and educate family members and caregivers about food allergies.

4. Emergency Preparedness: Develop an emergency action plan with healthcare providers to manage allergic reactions, including asthma exacerbations. Carry emergency medications like epinephrine auto-injectors, and educate close contacts on their use.

5. Monitor Symptoms: Regularly monitor asthma symptoms and food intake to identify potential triggers. Maintain a food diary to track reactions and share this information with healthcare providers.

6. Medical Alert: Wear a medical alert bracelet or carry a card indicating food allergies and asthma status, especially if at risk of severe allergic reactions.

7. Education and Support: Educate yourself and others about managing food allergies and asthma. Join support groups or seek guidance from healthcare professionals to enhance understanding and coping strategies.

8. Treatment Options: Discuss treatment options with healthcare providers, including medications to manage asthma symptoms and emergency treatments for severe allergic reactions. Immunotherapy may be considered for specific food allergies under medical supervision.

Conclusion

Food allergies pose a significant challenge for individuals with asthma, potentially worsening respiratory symptoms and complicating management. Understanding the interplay between food allergies and asthma, recognizing common allergens, and implementing effective management strategies are essential for achieving optimal respiratory health. By working closely with healthcare providers, avoiding allergenic foods, and preparing for emergencies, individuals with asthma can mitigate the impact of food allergies and lead a healthy, active life. Early recognition and proactive management of food allergies are pivotal in overcoming the challenges posed by asthma, ensuring improved quality of life for individuals and their families.

CHAPTER 9: MANAGING EXERCISE AND EMOTIONAL HEALTH

Managing asthma extends beyond medication and allergen avoidance; it includes maintaining a healthy lifestyle that incorporates regular exercise and emotional well-being. This chapter explores the importance of exercise for individuals with asthma, safe strategies for physical activity, and the impact of emotional health on asthma management.

Benefits of Exercise for Asthma

Regular exercise offers numerous advantages for individuals with asthma:

1. Improved Lung Function: Physical activity strengthens respiratory muscles and enhances lung function, facilitating easier breathing over time.

2. Enhanced Fitness: Regular exercise boosts overall fitness levels, making daily activities less demanding for those with asthma.

3. Weight Management: Maintaining a healthy weight through exercise reduces strain on the respiratory system and enhances asthma control.

4. Stress Reduction: Exercise helps alleviate stress, a common trigger for asthma symptoms in some individuals.

5. Improved Mood: Physical activity releases endorphins, fostering a positive mood and reducing feelings of anxiety and depression often associated with chronic conditions like asthma.

Safe Exercise Strategies for Asthmatics

While exercise is beneficial, individuals with asthma should take precautions to minimize the risk of triggering symptoms:

1. Warm-Up and Cool Down: Always warm up before exercising and cool down afterward to prepare the body and prevent abrupt changes in breathing patterns.

2. Choose Asthma-Friendly Activities: Opt for activities less likely to trigger asthma symptoms, such as swimming, walking, cycling, or yoga. Avoid activities involving prolonged exposure to cold, dry air, or high levels of pollen or pollution.

3. Use Asthma Medication as Directed: Take prescribed asthma medications as directed, especially before exercise, to prevent exercise-induced bronchoconstriction (EIB).

4. Monitor Breathing: Pay attention to breathing patterns during exercise. If experiencing wheezing, chest tightness, or shortness of breath, take a break and use a quick-relief inhaler as prescribed.

5. Stay Hydrated: Drink plenty of fluids before, during, and after exercise to keep airways hydrated and reduce the risk of asthma symptoms.

6. Be Aware of Weather Conditions: Exercise indoors on days with poor air quality or high pollen counts. In cold weather, use a scarf or mask over the nose and mouth to warm and humidify the air before breathing.

7. Inform Others: Notify exercise partners, coaches, or instructors about your asthma and emergency action plan in case of symptoms during physical activity.

Emotional Health and Asthma Management

Emotional well-being plays a vital role in asthma management, as stress and anxiety can exacerbate symptoms. Strategies to promote emotional health include:

1. Stress Management Techniques: Practice relaxation methods such as deep breathing, meditation, or yoga to reduce stress levels and minimize asthma triggers.

2. Cognitive Behavioral Therapy (CBT): CBT helps individuals with asthma identify and change negative thought patterns contributing to stress and anxiety, thereby improving asthma control.

3. Maintain a Support System: Build a support network of family, friends, and healthcare providers who understand and can assist with managing asthma and emotional health challenges.

4. Engage in Enjoyable Activities: Participate in hobbies and activities that bring joy and relaxation, promoting overall well-being and reducing stress.

5. Seek Professional Help: Consult mental health professionals or counselors if stress, anxiety, or depression related to asthma management becomes overwhelming.

Integrating Exercise and Emotional Health into Daily Life

To manage asthma effectively, incorporate regular exercise and emotional health strategies into daily routines:

1. Establish a Routine: Develop a consistent exercise schedule that includes warm-ups, cool-downs, and asthma-friendly activities. Aim for at least 30 minutes of moderate-intensity exercise most days of the week.

2. Set Realistic Goals: Set achievable fitness goals to gradually enhance physical fitness and asthma control.

Celebrate milestones to maintain motivation.

3. Monitor Asthma Symptoms: Keep track of symptoms, triggers, and medication use in a journal or app to identify patterns and adjust management strategies as needed.

4. Adapt to Challenges: Be flexible and adjust exercise plans based on asthma symptoms, weather conditions, and other factors affecting physical activity.

5. Prioritize Self-Care: Make self-care a priority by ensuring adequate sleep, a balanced diet, and regular exercise—all of which contribute to overall well-being and asthma management.

Conclusion

Managing asthma involves a holistic approach that includes medication adherence, allergen avoidance, regular exercise, and emotional well-being. By understanding the benefits of exercise, implementing safe strategies, and prioritizing emotional health, individuals with asthma can significantly improve respiratory function, reduce symptoms, and enhance overall quality of life. Effective asthma management requires finding balance, staying informed, and adapting lifestyle habits to support respiratory health and emotional well-being. With proactive management and a positive outlook, individuals can overcome the challenges posed by asthma and lead fulfilling, active lives.

CHAPTER 10: ADDRESSING CONCURRENT MEDICAL CONDITIONS

Living with asthma involves managing not only the respiratory symptoms but also addressing other medical conditions that frequently accompany it. This chapter explores common medical conditions that coexist with asthma, their impact on asthma management, and effective strategies for managing them.

Common Concurrent Medical Conditions

1. Allergic Rhinitis (Hay Fever):
   Allergic rhinitis often coexists with asthma due to shared airway inflammation. Triggers like pollen, dust mites, and pet dander can cause symptoms such as sneezing, runny nose, and nasal congestion, which exacerbate asthma. Managing allergic rhinitis involves allergen avoidance, medications like antihistamines and nasal sprays, and in severe cases, allergy shots.

2. Gastroesophageal Reflux Disease (GERD):
   GERD occurs when stomach acid backs up into the esophagus, causing

heartburn and potentially respiratory symptoms like coughing and wheezing. Acid reflux can irritate the airways, worsening asthma symptoms. Management strategies include lifestyle changes (e.g., dietary adjustments, elevating the head of the bed), medications to reduce acid production, and sometimes surgical interventions.

3. Obesity:

Obesity is associated with increased severity of asthma and poorer asthma control. Excess weight restricts lung expansion, leading to breathing difficulties and exacerbating asthma symptoms. Managing obesity through diet, exercise, and lifestyle changes can alleviate strain on the respiratory system and improve asthma outcomes.

4. Chronic Sinusitis:

Chronic sinus inflammation lasting over 12 weeks can trigger asthma exacerbations. Symptoms such as nasal congestion and sinus pressure contribute to mouth breathing, worsening asthma symptoms. Treatment options include nasal corticosteroids, saline rinses, antibiotics for bacterial infections, and sinus surgery in severe cases to improve sinus drainage.

5. Sleep Apnea:

Sleep apnea involves interrupted breathing during sleep, leading to decreased oxygen levels and daytime fatigue, which can exacerbate asthma symptoms. Continuous Positive Airway

Pressure (CPAP) therapy is the primary treatment to keep airways open and improve sleep quality, thereby reducing asthma exacerbations.

6. Anxiety and Depression:

Anxiety and depression are common among individuals with chronic conditions like asthma and can exacerbate symptoms through stress-induced mechanisms. Treatment options include therapy (e.g., cognitive-behavioral therapy), medications (e.g., antidepressants, anti-anxiety medications), and stress management techniques (e.g., relaxation exercises, mindfulness).

Impact of Concurrent Conditions on Asthma Management

Coexisting medical conditions complicate asthma management by:

- **Increasing Asthma Symptoms:** Conditions like allergic rhinitis, GERD, and sinusitis trigger or worsen asthma symptoms such as coughing, wheezing, and shortness of breath.

- **Reducing Asthma Control:** Obesity and sleep apnea impair lung function and decrease the effectiveness of asthma medications, leading to poorer asthma control.

- **Affecting Treatment Choices:** Some medications used to treat concurrent conditions may interact with asthma medications or exacerbate asthma symptoms. Coordinated treatment plans are essential to optimize outcomes.

- **Impacting Quality of Life:** Anxiety, depression, and chronic conditions affect overall well-being and adherence to asthma management strategies.

Strategies for Addressing Concurrent Medical Conditions

1. Comprehensive Assessment: Conduct a thorough medical evaluation to diagnose and manage concurrent conditions that impact asthma.

2. Integrated Treatment Plans: Develop coordinated treatment plans involving collaboration between healthcare providers specializing in asthma, allergies, gastroenterology, sleep medicine, and mental health.

3. Medication Management: Ensure medications prescribed for concurrent conditions are compatible with asthma treatments and adjust dosages as needed to minimize adverse effects.

4. Lifestyle Modifications: Implement lifestyle changes such as weight management, dietary adjustments, smoking cessation, and improved sleep hygiene to support overall health and asthma control.

5. Patient Education: Educate patients about how concurrent conditions affect asthma symptoms and emphasize the importance of adhering to treatment plans.

6. Regular Monitoring: Monitor asthma symptoms, medication adherence, and concurrent condition management regularly to assess treatment effectiveness and adjust strategies as necessary.

Conclusion

Addressing concurrent medical conditions is crucial for effectively managing asthma and improving overall health outcomes. By identifying and treating conditions like allergic rhinitis, GERD, obesity, chronic sinusitis, sleep apnea, anxiety, and depression, individuals with asthma can achieve better symptom control, fewer exacerbations, and improved quality of life. Coordinated care involving various healthcare specialists ensures comprehensive management tailored to each patient's needs. With proactive management and personalized care, individuals can overcome the challenges associated with asthma and lead healthier, more fulfilling lives.

CHAPTER 11: ALLERGY TESTING AND IMMUNOTHERAPY

Allergy testing and immunotherapy are crucial strategies in the management of asthma, particularly when allergies are significant triggers or exacerbators of symptoms. This chapter explores the importance of allergy testing, outlines various testing methods available, and discusses how allergen immunotherapy can empower individuals to overcome the challenges posed by allergic asthma.

Understanding Allergic Asthma

Allergic asthma is a type of asthma triggered by allergens like pollen, dust mites, pet dander, mold, and certain foods. Exposure to these allergens prompts an exaggerated immune response, leading to inflammation in the airways and resulting in symptoms such as wheezing, coughing, chest tightness, and shortness of breath.

Identifying specific allergens through allergy testing is critical for developing effective management strategies, including allergen avoidance, medication choices, and potentially allergen immunotherapy.

Types of Allergy Testing

Several methods are used for allergy testing, each offering unique advantages and insights into allergen sensitivities:

1. Skin Prick Test (SPT):
   - Procedure: A small amount of allergen extract is pricked into the skin, typically on the forearm or back.
   - Results: Allergic reactions appear as small, raised bumps (wheals) surrounded by redness (flares) within 15-20 minutes for positive reactions.
   - Advantages: It's rapid, cost-effective, and provides immediate results for common allergens.

2. Blood Tests (RAST or Specific IgE Tests):

- Procedure: Blood is drawn and tested for specific IgE antibodies against allergens.
- Results: Results are usually available within a few days and offer quantitative data on allergen sensitivities.
- Advantages: Useful when skin testing isn't feasible or when skin conditions interfere with testing.

3. Patch Testing:

-Procedure: Small amounts of allergens are applied to the skin and covered with patches for 48 hours.
- Results: Used to diagnose contact dermatitis from delayed allergic reactions to substances like metals, fragrances, or preservatives.

- Advantages: Identifies allergens causing skin reactions rather than respiratory symptoms.

Role of Allergy Testing in Asthma Management

Allergy testing plays a pivotal role in asthma management by:

- **Identifying Triggers:** Pinpointing specific allergens that trigger asthma symptoms allows for targeted allergen avoidance strategies.

- **Guiding Treatment:** Results from allergy testing inform the use of medications such as antihistamines, nasal corticosteroids, and allergen immunotherapy.

- **Personalizing Immunotherapy:** Allergy testing helps determine the suitability of allergen immunotherapy (desensitization) and identifies which allergens to include in the treatment plan.

Allergen Immunotherapy (Allergy Shots)

Allergen immunotherapy, commonly known as allergy shots, is a treatment option for allergic asthma aimed at reducing sensitivity to allergens and mitigating the severity of allergic reactions over time. Here's how it operates:

- **Administration:** Allergy shots involve administering small amounts of allergens via regular injections, with doses gradually increased to build tolerance.

- **Mechanism:** By exposing the immune system to controlled allergen doses, immunotherapy modifies immune responses, thereby reducing allergic reactions and asthma symptoms.

- **Duration:** Treatment typically begins with a build-up phase, during which injections are given once or twice weekly. This is followed by a maintenance phase with less frequent injections (e.g., every 2-4 weeks).

- **Effectiveness:** Immunotherapy is effective in decreasing symptoms and reducing medication usage in many allergic asthma patients, offering sustained benefits even post-treatment.

Benefits of Allergen Immunotherapy

Allergen immunotherapy offers several advantages for individuals with allergic asthma:

1. Symptom Reduction: Immunotherapy diminishes the frequency and severity of asthma symptoms triggered by allergens.

2. Decreased Medication Dependency: Many patients

experience reduced reliance on asthma medications, including rescue inhalers and controller medications.

3. Long-term Relief: Immunotherapy provides enduring relief from allergy symptoms and asthma, extending beyond the treatment duration.

4. Preventative Effect: Some studies indicate that immunotherapy may prevent the onset of new allergies and asthma in children with allergic rhinitis.

Considerations for Allergen Immunotherapy

Before initiating allergen immunotherapy, it's essential to consider the following factors:

- **Patient Selection:** Immunotherapy is typically recommended for individuals with moderate to severe allergic asthma triggered by specific allergens identified through testing.

- **Safety:** While generally safe, allergen immunotherapy carries a risk of allergic reactions, necessitating administration under medical supervision.

- **Commitment:** Treatment requires regular visits to the allergist for injections, particularly during the build-up phase.

- **Duration:** Immunotherapy is a long-term commitment, requiring several years to achieve optimal results.

Conclusion

Allergy testing and immunotherapy are indispensable components of managing allergic asthma effectively. By identifying specific allergens through testing and undergoing allergen immunotherapy, individuals can significantly alleviate asthma symptoms, reduce medication usage, and enhance overall quality of life. Healthcare providers play a crucial role in tailoring treatment plans based on allergy test findings and closely monitoring progress to ensure favorable outcomes. With allergen immunotherapy, individuals with allergic asthma can break free from the constraints imposed by allergens and embrace a healthier, more active lifestyle.

In summary, allergy testing and immunotherapy are essential tools for effectively managing allergic asthma. By identifying allergens and undergoing desensitization through immunotherapy, individuals can mitigate asthma symptoms, minimize medication use, and achieve sustained relief. Healthcare providers' guidance is pivotal in navigating this process, ensuring personalized care plans and optimal outcomes. With commitment and comprehensive management, individuals can liberate themselves from the limitations of allergic asthma and pursue a healthier future.

CHAPTER 12: A DETAILED GUIDE TO ASTHMA MEDICATIONS

Asthma medications are pivotal for managing symptoms, preventing flare-ups, and enhancing the quality of life for asthma sufferers. This chapter provides an extensive overview of asthma medications, encompassing their types, functions, methods of administration, and key considerations for usage.

Understanding Asthma Medications

Asthma medications are broadly categorized into two main types: controller medications and quick-relief (rescue) medications, each serving distinct roles in managing asthma symptoms and maintaining optimal lung function.

Controller Medications

Controller medications are long-term treatments designed to reduce airway inflammation, prevent asthma symptoms, and minimize reliance on quick-relief medications. They are typically used daily, even during periods of symptom remission, to sustain lung function and prevent asthma exacerbations. Examples of controller medications include:

1. Inhaled Corticosteroids (ICS):
   - Function: ICS medications reduce airway inflammation, making the airways less sensitive to triggers.
   - Examples: Fluticasone (Flovent), Budesonide (Pulmicort), Beclomethasone (Qvar).
   - Administration: Administered via inhalers (metered-dose or dry powder inhalers).
   - Considerations: Effective when used consistently; rinsing the mouth after use helps prevent oral thrush.

2. Long-acting Beta-agonists (LABAs):

- Function: LABAs relax the smooth muscles around the airways, facilitating easier breathing.
- Examples: Salmeterol (Serevent), Formoterol (Foradil).
- Administration: Administered via inhalers; should not be used alone without an ICS.

3. Combination Inhalers:

- Function: These inhalers contain both an ICS and a LABA, offering anti-inflammatory and bronchodilator effects.
- Examples: Fluticasone/Salmeterol (Advair), Budesonide/Formoterol (Symbicort).
- Administration: Available as metered-dose or dry powder inhalers.

4. Leukotriene Modifiers:

- Function: Block the action of leukotrienes, substances that cause inflammation and airway constriction.
- Examples: Montelukast (Singulair), Zafirlukast (Accolate).
- Administration: Oral tablets or chewable tablets; often used in conjunction with ICS.

5. Mast Cell Stabilizers:

- Function: Stabilize mast cells in the airways, reducing the release of inflammatory substances.
- Examples: Cromolyn (Intal), Nedocromil (Tilade).
- Administration: Administered via inhalers (less common) or nebulizers.

6. Biologics:

- Function: Target specific immune pathways involved in allergic asthma.

- Examples: Omalizumab (Xolair), Mepolizumab (Nucala), Dupilumab (Dupixent).

- Administration: Given via subcutaneous injections or intravenous infusions; reserved for severe asthma cases.

Quick-Relief (Rescue) Medications

Quick-relief medications provide rapid relief during asthma attacks or exacerbations by relaxing the muscles around the airways. They include:

1. Short-acting Beta-agonists (SABAs):
   - Function: Quickly relax airway muscles, easing breathing.
   - Examples: Albuterol (Ventolin), Levalbuterol (Xopenex).
   - Administration: Administered via metered-dose inhalers, nebulizers, or occasionally as oral tablets.

2. Anticholinergics (Short-acting):
   - Function: Help relax airway muscles and reduce mucus production.
   - Examples: Ipratropium (Atrovent).
   - Administration: Administered via inhalers or nebulizers.

Considerations for Asthma Medication Use

Effective asthma management involves several considerations when selecting and using medications:

- **Personalized Treatment Plans:** Tailor medications based on individual asthma severity, triggers, and treatment response.

- **Medication Delivery Devices:** Proper inhaler or nebulizer technique is critical for medication efficacy. Patients should receive thorough education on correct usage.

- **Potential Side Effects:** All asthma medications carry potential side effects, from mild (e.g., oral thrush with ICS) to severe (e.g., cardiac effects with LABAs). Regular monitoring and communication with healthcare providers are essential.

- **Adherence to Treatment:** Consistent use of controller medications, even during symptom-free periods, is crucial for preventing exacerbations and maintaining lung function.

- **Emergency Action Plans:** Patients should have a written asthma action plan outlining steps for managing worsening symptoms or asthma attacks, including when to use quick-relief medications and when to seek medical help.

Managing Asthma with Medications

Optimal asthma control requires proactive medication management:

1. Regular Monitoring: Healthcare providers should monitor asthma symptoms, lung function tests (e.g., peak flow measurements), and medication adherence during routine visits.

2. Adjusting Treatment: Medication doses may need adjustment based on changes in asthma severity, triggers, or overall health.

3. Patient Education: Educating patients about asthma medications, their purposes, correct usage techniques, and potential side effects improves adherence and treatment outcomes.

4. Lifestyle Management:
Encouraging lifestyle changes such as smoking cessation, regular exercise, and allergen avoidance complements medication therapy in enhancing asthma control.

Conclusion

Asthma medications are essential for effectively managing symptoms, preventing exacerbations, and improving overall quality of life. By understanding the types of medications available, proper administration techniques, and personalized treatment plans, individuals with asthma can collaborate with healthcare providers to develop strategies that meet their specific needs. Through adherence to prescribed medications, effective communication with healthcare providers, and proactive management, individuals can effectively manage asthma and lead healthier lives.

In summary, asthma medications are pivotal in managing symptoms and enhancing quality of life. With a comprehensive grasp of medication types, correct usage techniques, and personalized treatment plans, individuals can successfully control their asthma and minimize its impact on daily life. Healthcare providers play a crucial role in guiding medication choices, ensuring optimal asthma management, and empowering individuals to achieve long-term asthma control.

CHAPTER 13: UNDERSTANDING ASTHMA CONTROLLER MEDICATIONS

Asthma controller medications are indispensable tools for effectively managing asthma, alleviating symptoms, and preventing exacerbations. This chapter aims to provide a comprehensive understanding of asthma controller medications, covering their types, functions, methods of administration, considerations for usage, and the crucial role of adherence in achieving optimal asthma control.

Types of Asthma Controller Medications

Asthma controller medications are designed for long-term use to manage the underlying inflammation in the airways, thereby reducing the frequency and severity of asthma symptoms. These medications are typically used daily, even when asthma symptoms are well-managed, to sustain lung function and prevent flare-ups. The main categories of asthma controller medications include:

1. Inhaled Corticosteroids (ICS)

-Function: Inhaled corticosteroids are the most commonly prescribed controller medications for asthma. They work by reducing inflammation in the airways, making them less sensitive to triggers like allergens and irritants.

-Examples: Commonly prescribed ICS medications include Fluticasone (Flovent), Budesonide (Pulmicort), Beclomethasone (Qvar), and Ciclesonide (Alvesco).

-Administration: ICS medications are delivered directly to the lungs via inhalers, which can be metered-dose inhalers (MDIs) or dry powder inhalers (DPIs). Proper inhaler technique is crucial for effective medication delivery.

-Considerations: It is advisable to rinse the mouth after using ICS inhalers to prevent potential side effects such as oral thrush.

2. Long-acting Beta-agonists (LABAs)

-Function: Long-acting beta-agonists help relax the smooth muscles around the airways, making it easier to breathe. They are often used in combination with ICS medications to provide both anti-inflammatory and bronchodilator effects.

-Examples: Salmeterol (Serevent) and Formoterol (Foradil) are commonly used LABAs in asthma management.

-Administration: LABAs are administered through inhalers and should never be used as monotherapy for asthma. They are always combined with an ICS to achieve optimal asthma control.

3. Combination Inhalers (ICS/LABA)

-Function: Combination inhalers contain both an inhaled corticosteroid and a long-acting beta-agonist in a single device. They offer the benefits of anti-inflammatory action from ICS and bronchodilation from LABAs.

-Examples: Well-known combination inhalers include Advair (Fluticasone/Salmeterol), Symbicort (Budesonide/Formoterol), and Dulera (Mometasone/Formoterol).

-Administration: Available as metered-dose inhalers (MDIs) or dry powder inhalers (DPIs), combination inhalers simplify medication regimens by delivering two types of medication in one inhaler.

4. Leukotriene Modifiers

-Function: Leukotriene modifiers block the action of leukotrienes, inflammatory substances that contribute to asthma symptoms and airway constriction.

-Examples: Montelukast (Singulair), Zafirlukast (Accolate), and Zileuton (Zyflo) are oral medications categorized under this class.

-Administration: Leukotriene modifiers are typically available as tablets or chewable tablets, taken once daily. They may be prescribed as adjunct therapy to ICS when additional symptom control is necessary.

5. Mast Cell Stabilizers

-Function: Mast cell stabilizers prevent the release of inflammatory substances from mast cells in the airways, thereby reducing the likelihood of asthma attacks triggered by allergens or exercise.

-Examples: Cromolyn (Intal) and Nedocromil (Tilade) are examples of mast cell stabilizers.

-Administration: Historically administered via inhalers, mast cell stabilizers are less commonly used today but remain available in some regions for specific asthma management needs.

6. Biologics

-Function: Biologic medications target specific immune pathways involved in allergic asthma. They are reserved for severe asthma cases that do not respond well to traditional treatments.

-Examples: Omalizumab (Xolair), Mepolizumab (Nucala), Reslizumab

(Cinqair), and Benralizumab (Fasenra) are biologics approved for asthma treatment.

-Administration: Biologics are administered via subcutaneous injections or intravenous infusions at specified intervals. Due to their targeted effects on the immune system, they require careful monitoring.

Benefits of Asthma Controller Medications

Asthma controller medications provide several advantages in the management of asthma:
- **Reduced Inflammation:** By targeting airway inflammation, these medications

help prevent the underlying causes of asthma symptoms.

- Improved Symptom Control: Regular use of controller medications reduces the frequency and severity of asthma attacks, allowing individuals to lead more active lives.

- Prevention of Exacerbations: By maintaining stable lung function, these medications minimize the risk of asthma exacerbations that may necessitate emergency medical intervention.

- Long-term Lung Protection: Effective use of controller medications can slow the progression of asthma and reduce the likelihood of developing irreversible lung damage over time.

Considerations for Using Asthma Controller Medications

While highly effective, the successful use of asthma controller medications requires careful consideration of several factors:

- **Adherence:** Consistent daily use of controller medications, even during periods of symptom relief, is crucial for achieving optimal asthma control.

- **Monitoring and Adjustment:** Healthcare providers should regularly monitor asthma symptoms and lung function to adjust medication doses as necessary based on individual response and changing asthma severity.

- Side Effects: Like all medications, asthma controller medications may have potential side effects. Patients should be aware of these and promptly report any concerns to their healthcare provider.

- Individualized Treatment Plans: Asthma management should be personalized to each patient's specific needs, considering factors such as asthma severity, triggers, comorbid conditions, and medication preferences.

Conclusion

Asthma controller medications play a critical role in maintaining stable lung function, reducing inflammation, and preventing asthma attacks. By understanding the various types of controller medications available, how they work, and the considerations for their use, individuals with asthma can collaborate effectively with healthcare providers to develop tailored treatment plans that optimize asthma control and enhance overall quality of life.

In summary, asthma controller medications are essential tools for managing asthma effectively, reducing symptoms, and improving long-term lung health. Through adherence to prescribed medications, regular monitoring, and open communication with healthcare providers, individuals can effectively manage asthma and overcome the challenges associated with this chronic respiratory condition.

CHAPTER 14: EFFECTIVE MANAGEMENT OF ASTHMA EPISODES

Asthma episodes, also known as asthma attacks or exacerbations, can be frightening and potentially life-threatening if not promptly and effectively managed. This chapter offers essential guidance on identifying asthma symptoms, understanding the stages of an asthma attack, and outlining the steps necessary to treat asthma episodes effectively, thereby regaining control and preventing complications.

Recognizing Asthma Symptoms

Recognizing the early signs and symptoms of asthma is critical for initiating timely treatment and preventing the escalation of an asthma episode. Common symptoms include:

- **Shortness of breath:** Difficulty breathing, rapid breathing, or feeling unable to take in enough air.
- **Wheezing:** High-pitched whistling sounds while breathing out, often noticeable during exhalation.
- **Coughing:** Persistent cough, particularly worse at night or early in the morning.
- **Chest tightness:** Sensation of pressure or constriction in the chest.

- **Increased mucus production:** Production of thick, sticky mucus in the airways.
- **Fatigue:** Feeling tired or weak due to the effort required to breathe.

Stages of an Asthma Attack

Understanding the stages of an asthma attack is crucial for individuals and caregivers to respond effectively and seek appropriate medical assistance when necessary:

1. Early Warning Signs:

- Subtle symptoms: Mild coughing, occasional wheezing, or slight shortness of breath.

- Response: Taking action at this stage can prevent symptoms from progressing into a full-blown asthma attack.

2. Mild to Moderate Symptoms:

- Increased symptoms: Persistent cough, wheezing with each breath, moderate shortness of breath.
- Action: Use of quick-relief medications (rescue inhalers) to alleviate symptoms. Continuous monitoring for any signs of worsening is essential.

3. Severe Symptoms:

- Intense symptoms: Severe shortness of breath, extreme wheezing, difficulty speaking in full sentences, tightness in the chest.

- Emergency: Immediate administration of quick-relief medications is crucial. Contacting emergency services or visiting the nearest healthcare facility is necessary if symptoms do not improve within minutes or if they worsen.

Steps for Effective Treatment of Asthma Episodes

Prompt and appropriate treatment of asthma episodes can prevent complications and minimize the need for emergency interventions. Here are the recommended steps for effectively treating asthma episodes:

Step 1: Assess Symptom Severity

- Evaluate symptoms: Assess the severity of asthma symptoms (mild, moderate, or severe) to determine the appropriate treatment approach.
- Use of peak flow meter: If available, measure the peak expiratory flow rate (PEFR) to monitor lung function and gauge the severity of the episode.

Step 2: Use Quick-Relief Medications (Rescue Inhalers)

- Administer bronchodilators: Use quick-relief medications such as short-acting beta-agonists (SABA) like albuterol to relax the muscles around the airways, facilitating improved airflow.

- Adherence to dosage: Administer the medication according to the prescribed or healthcare provider's instructions. Repeat doses as necessary based on symptom severity and response.

Step 3: Implement Breathing Techniques

- Practice controlled breathing: Encourage slow, deep breaths to help relax and open up the airways, easing breathing difficulties.
- Positioning: Sit upright or in a comfortable position that supports easier breathing.

Step 4: Monitor Response and Seek Medical Assistance

- Monitor symptoms: Continuously monitor the response to medication and watch for any signs of symptom worsening.
- Contact healthcare provider: If symptoms persist or worsen despite medication use, seek immediate medical attention or contact emergency services.

Step 5: Follow Asthma Action Plan

- Refer to asthma action plan: Follow the personalized asthma action plan developed with healthcare providers to guide treatment during asthma episodes.

- Adjust medication: Make adjustments to medication doses as recommended in the action plan to manage worsening symptoms or exacerbations effectively.

Step 6: Preventive Measures and Aftercare

- Identify triggers: Identify and avoid triggers that may have triggered the asthma episode to prevent future occurrences.
- Review and follow-up: Schedule follow-up appointments with healthcare providers to review asthma management strategies and make any necessary adjustments to the treatment plan.
- Self-care: Rest, stay hydrated, and avoid strenuous activities until symptoms improve. Use a peak flow

meter if advised by healthcare providers to monitor lung function.

Conclusion

Effectively managing asthma episodes involves timely recognition of symptoms, prompt use of quick-relief medications, and adherence to personalized asthma action plans. By understanding the stages of an asthma attack and implementing appropriate treatment strategies, individuals can regain control over their respiratory health and minimize the impact of asthma on daily life.

In summary, treating asthma episodes effectively requires proactive management, adherence to prescribed medications, and readiness to seek medical assistance when necessary. Empowering individuals with knowledge and tools to respond promptly to asthma symptoms aims to support better asthma control and enhance the quality of life for individuals living with asthma.

CHAPTER 15: ASTHMA IN CHILDREN AND ADOLESCENTS

Asthma stands as one of the most prevalent chronic conditions affecting children and adolescents globally. Understanding how asthma manifests in younger individuals, along with effective management strategies and the unique challenges they encounter, is crucial for improving treatment outcomes and enhancing their quality of life. This chapter provides essential insights into asthma among children and adolescents, covering its prevalence, symptoms, diagnosis, treatment options, and practical advice for parents and caregivers.

Prevalence of Asthma in Children and Adolescents

Asthma impacts approximately 5-10% of children worldwide, making it one of the most widespread chronic diseases in pediatric populations. It can onset at any age, and symptoms vary in intensity and frequency among individuals. Timely diagnosis and proactive management play pivotal roles in controlling symptoms and averting exacerbations that can disrupt a child's daily activities and overall well-being.

Symptoms of Asthma in Children and Adolescents

Identifying asthma symptoms in children and adolescents poses challenges due to variations compared to adults. Common symptoms include:

- **Coughing:** Persistent cough, particularly noticeable at night or early morning.
- **Wheezing:** High-pitched whistling sounds during exhalation.
- Shortness of breath: Difficulty breathing, rapid breathing, or sensations of chest tightness.
- **Chest tightness:** Feeling pressure or discomfort in the chest area.
- **Fatigue:** Feelings of tiredness or weakness due to respiratory difficulties.

- Reduced physical activity: Reluctance to engage in physical activities due to breathlessness.

Symptoms may fluctuate over time, with periods of exacerbation (asthma attacks) interspersed with periods of remission. Vigilant monitoring by parents and caregivers is essential, with prompt medical attention advised if concerns arise about asthma or related respiratory issues.

Diagnosis of Asthma in Children and Adolescents

Diagnosing asthma in younger individuals involves a comprehensive approach incorporating medical history, physical examinations, and diagnostic tests. Key considerations include:

- **Medical history:** Thorough assessment of symptoms, triggers, and family history of asthma or allergies.
- **Physical examination:** Evaluation of respiratory function, including lung sounds and breathing patterns.
- **Diagnostic tests:** Utilization of pulmonary function tests (spirometry) and allergy testing to assess lung function and identify potential triggers.

Diagnostic criteria may vary based on the child's age, symptoms, and medical background. Collaborative efforts between healthcare providers, parents, and caregivers are crucial in establishing an accurate diagnosis and formulating a personalized treatment plan.

Treatment Options for Asthma in Children and Adolescents

The management of asthma in children and adolescents centers on symptom control, prevention of exacerbations, and support for normal physical activities and development. Treatment options encompass:

1. Controller Medications

- Inhaled corticosteroids (ICS): Mitigate airway inflammation and prevent symptoms when used regularly.

- Long-acting beta-agonists (LABAs): Provide bronchodilation and are often combined with ICS for enhanced asthma management.
- Leukotriene modifiers: Block inflammatory substances contributing to asthma symptoms.

Prescription of controller medications is based on asthma severity and the child's response to treatment. Strict adherence to medication schedules is vital for maintaining asthma control and reducing the risk of complications.

2. Quick-Relief Medications

- Short-acting beta-agonists (SABAs): Administered during asthma attacks to swiftly relieve bronchospasm and improve breathing.

Parents and caregivers should ensure that quick-relief medications are readily accessible and used as directed during exacerbations or worsening symptoms.

3. Allergy Management

- Allergen avoidance: Identification and minimization of exposure to triggers such as dust mites, pet dander, pollen, and mold.
- Allergy medications: Administration of antihistamines or allergy shots (immunotherapy) may be recommended for children with allergic asthma.

Effective management of allergies aids in reducing asthma symptoms and enhancing overall respiratory health in children and adolescents.

Practical Tips for Parents and Caregivers

Supporting a child or adolescent with asthma necessitates proactive management and the creation of an environment conducive to respiratory health:

- **Education:** Acquire knowledge about asthma symptoms, triggers, medications, and emergency response protocols.
- **Asthma action plan:** Develop a personalized asthma action plan with healthcare providers outlining daily medications, asthma triggers, symptom

management strategies, and emergency contacts.

- **Symptom monitoring:** Regularly track asthma symptoms, peak flow readings (if applicable), and medication adherence.

- **Encouraging physical activity:** Foster participation in suitable physical activities while ensuring asthma medications are readily available if needed.

- **Promoting a healthy environment:** Maintain clean indoor air quality, minimize exposure to tobacco smoke, and reduce allergens that may trigger asthma symptoms.

Conclusion

Asthma management in children and adolescents necessitates a comprehensive approach that addresses symptoms, triggers, and personalized treatment plans to achieve optimal asthma control. By comprehending the distinct challenges and implementing effective management strategies, parents and caregivers can effectively support children with asthma and enhance their overall well-being.

In summary, early diagnosis, proactive treatment, and ongoing support are critical for managing asthma in children and adolescents. By collaborating closely with healthcare providers and implementing practical strategies, parents and caregivers empower young individuals with asthma to lead active, healthy lives, overcoming the limitations imposed by this chronic respiratory condition.

CHAPTER 16: ASTHMA MANAGEMENT DURING PREGNANCY

Managing asthma during pregnancy is crucial for ensuring both maternal health and the optimal development of the fetus. This chapter delves into the unique challenges of asthma management during pregnancy, explores safe treatment options, discusses potential risks, and provides practical advice for pregnant individuals with asthma.

Understanding Asthma During Pregnancy

Asthma is a chronic respiratory condition characterized by airway inflammation, leading to symptoms like wheezing, breathlessness, chest tightness, and coughing. Pregnancy introduces additional complexities due to hormonal changes, altered immune responses, and physical transformations, all of which can influence asthma symptoms and their management.

Prevalence and Impact

Approximately 4-8% of pregnant individuals experience asthma, with variations based on individual health factors and environmental triggers.

Effectively managing asthma during pregnancy is critical because uncontrolled asthma can increase risks for both the mother and the developing fetus:

- **Maternal risks:** Elevated chances of conditions like preeclampsia, gestational diabetes, and worsening asthma symptoms.
- **Fetal risks:** Higher incidences of preterm birth, low birth weight, and potential developmental issues if maternal oxygen levels are compromised during severe asthma episodes.

Safe Treatment Options

The management of asthma during pregnancy revolves around balancing the need for symptom control with the safety of treatments for both mother and baby. Key considerations include:

1. Controller Medications

- Inhaled corticosteroids (ICS): Preferred as the first-line treatment during pregnancy for their ability to reduce airway inflammation with minimal systemic absorption.
- Long-acting beta-agonists (LABAs): Used in combination with ICS if additional bronchodilation is necessary.

2. Quick-Relief Medications

- Short-acting beta-agonists (SABAs)' Rescue medications that provide immediate relief during asthma exacerbations and are considered safe throughout pregnancy when used as prescribed.

3. Avoidance of Triggers

- Identification and minimization: Efforts to reduce exposure to allergens and irritants such as dust mites, pet dander, smoke, and environmental pollutants.

4. Regular Monitoring and Healthcare Consultation

- Asthma action plan: Develop a personalized plan with healthcare providers outlining daily medications, strategies for managing symptoms, and steps to take during exacerbations.
- Routine check-ups: Attend scheduled prenatal visits and asthma check-ups to

monitor asthma control, fetal development, and adjust treatment plans as needed.

Risks and Considerations

While many asthma medications are generally considered safe during pregnancy, there are specific considerations and potential risks:

- **Oral corticosteroids:** Long-term use may increase the risk of conditions like gestational diabetes, hypertension, and low birth weight. They are typically reserved for severe exacerbations when benefits outweigh risks.

- **Certain medications:** Drugs such as leukotriene modifiers and theophylline have limited safety data during pregnancy and are usually avoided unless deemed necessary by healthcare providers.
- **Fetal monitoring:** Regular ultrasound examinations may be recommended, especially if asthma symptoms are severe or poorly controlled, to monitor fetal growth and development.

Practical Tips for Asthma Management During Pregnancy

Effective management of asthma during pregnancy involves proactive steps and vigilance. Here are practical tips for pregnant individuals with asthma:

- **Adherence to medication:** Follow prescribed medication schedules rigorously to maintain asthma control.
- **Trigger avoidance:** Minimize exposure to known triggers to prevent asthma symptoms from worsening.
- **Healthy lifestyle:** Maintain a balanced diet, engage in moderate physical activity as advised, and avoid smoking and secondhand smoke.
- **Adequate hydration:** Ensure sufficient water intake to keep respiratory passages hydrated, potentially easing asthma symptoms.
- **Rest and stress management:** Prioritize adequate rest and practice relaxation techniques like deep

breathing exercises to manage stress, which can impact asthma symptoms.

Conclusion

Managing asthma during pregnancy necessitates collaboration between pregnant individuals, healthcare providers, and obstetric specialists to ensure the best outcomes for both mother and baby. By understanding the unique challenges, safe treatment options, and proactive management strategies, pregnant individuals with asthma can effectively control their symptoms and minimize the risk of complications.

In summary, maintaining asthma control during pregnancy involves carefully balancing medication safety with symptom management, avoiding triggers, and maintaining regular medical supervision. With proper care and adherence to treatment plans, pregnant individuals with asthma can navigate this period confidently, focusing on their health and the well-being of their developing baby.

CHAPTER 17: ASTHMA CHALLENGES IN THE ELDERLY

Asthma is commonly associated with children and younger adults, but it also presents distinctive challenges in older individuals. This chapter explores the unique aspects of asthma in the elderly population, covering its prevalence, symptoms, diagnosis, treatment considerations, and practical management strategies.

Prevalence of Asthma in Older Adults

Asthma is prevalent among older adults but often goes unrecognized or misdiagnosed due to symptoms that overlap with other respiratory conditions common in aging populations. Research indicates that approximately 5-10% of adults aged 65 and older are affected by asthma, although this figure varies based on location and demographics.

Symptoms experienced by older adults with asthma may differ from those seen in younger individuals:

- **Chronic cough:** Persistent coughing, often exacerbated at night.

- **Shortness of breath:** Difficulty breathing, especially during physical exertion.
- **Chest tightness:** Sensation of pressure or discomfort in the chest.
- **Wheezing:** High-pitched whistling sounds during exhalation.

Challenges in Diagnosing Asthma in Older Adults

Diagnosing asthma in older adults poses challenges due to several factors:

- **Symptom overlap:** Asthma symptoms can mimic those of chronic obstructive pulmonary disease (COPD), heart disease, or natural respiratory changes associated with aging.

- **Atypical presentation:** Older adults may present with fewer classic symptoms such as wheezing, making diagnosis more complex.
- **Comorbidities:** The presence of multiple chronic conditions complicates the diagnostic process.

Healthcare providers rely on a thorough medical history, physical examination, and pulmonary function tests like spirometry to distinguish asthma from other respiratory conditions in older adults.

Symptom Management and Treatment Considerations

Effective management of asthma in older adults involves addressing symptoms while considering age-related changes, comorbidities, and potential interactions with other medications. Treatment options include:

1. Controller Medications

- Inhaled corticosteroids (ICS): These medications reduce airway inflammation and are typically the first-line treatment for persistent asthma in older adults.

- Long-acting beta-agonists (LABAs): They provide additional bronchodilation and are sometimes used in combination with ICS.

2. Quick-Relief Medications

- Short-acting beta-agonists (SABAs): These medications provide rapid relief during asthma exacerbations.

3. Comprehensive Asthma Management

- Individualized treatment plans: Tailored to the severity of asthma, presence of comorbidities, and response to medications.
- Regular follow-up: Monitoring asthma control, adjusting medications as needed, and educating older adults

and caregivers on symptom management and adherence to medication regimens.

Practical Management Strategies for Older Adults with Asthma

Managing asthma effectively in older adults requires a holistic approach that addresses both medical and lifestyle factors. Practical strategies include:

- **Medication adherence:** Encouraging adherence to prescribed regimens and educating on proper inhaler techniques.
- **Comprehensive health management:** Coordinating care to address asthma alongside other chronic

conditions, ensuring medication compatibility and minimizing side effects.
- **Routine monitoring:** Regular assessment of symptoms, lung function, and potential triggers like allergies or environmental pollutants.
- **Health promotion:** Promoting a healthy lifestyle including balanced nutrition, appropriate physical activity, and smoking cessation if relevant.
- **Environmental control:** Minimizing exposure to allergens and irritants that can trigger asthma symptoms.

Unique Considerations and Challenges

Older adults with asthma face specific challenges that require tailored care:

- **Polypharmacy:** Managing multiple medications requires careful consideration to avoid interactions and adverse effects.
- **Cognitive and physical limitations:** Addressing challenges related to cognitive decline, mobility issues, and difficulties with inhaler use.
- **End-of-life planning:** Discussions about preferences for asthma management in the context of overall health and quality of life goals.

Conclusion

Asthma in older adults is a complex but manageable condition that necessitates a nuanced approach to diagnosis, treatment, and ongoing care. By recognizing the unique challenges, understanding treatment considerations, and implementing practical strategies, healthcare providers and caregivers can help older adults maintain asthma control and improve their quality of life.

In summary, effective asthma management in older adults requires collaboration among healthcare providers, caregivers, and older individuals themselves to customize treatment plans, optimize medication use, and address age-related concerns. With proper support and management, older adults with asthma can lead active, fulfilling lives while effectively managing their respiratory health.

CHAPTER 18: ADDITIONAL CONSIDERATIONS FOR ASTHMA

Asthma, a complex respiratory condition that varies greatly among individuals, necessitates careful consideration of various factors beyond basic diagnosis and treatment. This chapter explores additional aspects crucial for effectively managing asthma, including environmental influences, mental health impacts, alternative therapies, and advancements in research.

Environmental Factors Affecting Asthma

Environmental triggers play a pivotal role in triggering asthma symptoms and exacerbations. It is essential to understand and mitigate these influences for effective asthma management:

- **Indoor allergens:** Common triggers like dust mites, pet dander, mold, and cockroach droppings can significantly worsen asthma symptoms. Strategies such as regular cleaning routines, using allergen-proof bedding, and maintaining optimal humidity levels can help reduce exposure.

-**Outdoor pollutants:** Factors such as air pollution, pollen, and industrial emissions can also exacerbate asthma. Monitoring air quality forecasts, avoiding outdoor activities during high-pollution periods, and employing air purifiers indoors can mitigate these risks.

- **Weather conditions:** Cold air, humidity changes, and thunderstorms are known triggers for asthma attacks. Protective measures such as wearing scarves over the nose and mouth in cold weather and staying indoors during thunderstorms can reduce the likelihood of exacerbations.

Mental Health and Asthma

The relationship between asthma and mental health is complex and bidirectional, with each influencing the other:

- **Stress and anxiety:** Emotional stress can trigger asthma symptoms or make existing symptoms worse. Techniques such as deep breathing exercises, meditation, and yoga can effectively manage stress and alleviate asthma symptoms.

- **Depression:** The chronic nature of asthma may increase the risk of depression. Seeking support from mental health professionals and participating in support groups can provide emotional support and improve overall well-being.

Alternative Therapies for Asthma Management

Complementary and alternative therapies offer additional avenues for managing asthma, although their effectiveness varies widely:

- **Acupuncture:** This traditional Chinese practice involves inserting thin needles into specific points on the body to alleviate symptoms and promote overall health.

- **Herbal supplements:** Certain herbs such as Boswellia, Butterbur, and Ginger have anti-inflammatory properties that may help reduce asthma symptoms. It is crucial to consult healthcare providers before incorporating herbal supplements into treatment plans due to potential interactions with medications.

- **Breathing exercises:** Techniques like pursed-lip breathing and diaphragmatic breathing can enhance lung function and reduce the frequency of asthma attacks. These exercises are often taught in pulmonary rehabilitation programs or by qualified respiratory therapists.

Advances in Research and Treatment

Ongoing research continues to expand our understanding of asthma and introduce innovative treatment options:

- **Biological therapies:** Monoclonal antibodies targeting specific immune pathways have demonstrated effectiveness in treating severe asthma resistant to traditional therapies.

- **Gene therapy:** Research is underway to explore genetic factors contributing to asthma susceptibility and develop gene-based treatments.

- **Precision medicine:** Tailoring asthma treatment based on individual genetic and environmental factors aims to optimize treatment outcomes and minimize side effects.

Integrative Approaches to Asthma Management

Integrative medicine integrates conventional medical treatments with complementary therapies to address the comprehensive needs of asthma patients:

- **Holistic assessment:** Integrative healthcare providers conduct thorough evaluations considering physical, emotional, and environmental factors influencing asthma.

- **Personalized treatment plans:** Treatment plans are customized based on asthma severity, individual responses to medications, and lifestyle factors. This may include a combination of medications, dietary adjustments, stress management techniques, and alternative therapies.

- **Patient empowerment:** Encouraging individuals to actively engage in their asthma management empowers them to make informed decisions about their health and treatment options.

Conclusion

Effective asthma management goes beyond standard medical treatments to encompass environmental considerations, mental health support, alternative therapies, and ongoing advancements in research. By addressing these additional aspects, healthcare providers and individuals with asthma can improve treatment outcomes and enhance quality of life.

In summary, a comprehensive approach to asthma care involves understanding and mitigating environmental triggers, addressing mental health needs, exploring complementary therapies, staying updated on research advancements, and embracing integrative healthcare practices. By integrating these considerations into asthma management plans, individuals can overcome the challenges of their condition and achieve optimal respiratory health.

CHAPTER 19: ADVOCATING FOR YOURSELF AND OTHERS WITH ASTHMA

Advocacy plays a pivotal role in empowering individuals living with asthma to manage their condition effectively, access appropriate care, and raise awareness within their communities. This chapter explores the significance of self-advocacy, strategies for supporting others with asthma, and ways to contribute to broader advocacy efforts.

The Importance of Self-Advocacy

Self-advocacy entails actively advocating for oneself to ensure needs are met, rights are respected, and quality of care is optimized. For individuals coping with asthma, self-advocacy is essential for:

- **Accessing suitable care:** Clearly communicating symptoms, treatment preferences, and concerns to healthcare providers.

-**Navigating healthcare systems:** Understanding insurance coverage, medication costs, and available support services.

- **Enhancing treatment outcomes:** Taking an active role in treatment decisions, adherence, and monitoring asthma control.

Effective Strategies for Self-Advocacy

Empowering individuals with asthma to advocate for themselves involves practical approaches:

1. Educational empowerment: Acquiring knowledge about asthma symptoms, triggers, treatments, and self-management strategies to make informed decisions.

2. Communication proficiency: Articulating symptoms, treatment goals, and concerns clearly to healthcare providers. Asking questions and seeking clarification ensures effective communication.

3. Record keeping: Maintaining detailed records of asthma symptoms, medication usage, triggers, and healthcare interactions aids in tracking progress and facilitating productive medical appointments.

4. Understanding rights: Familiarizing oneself with healthcare entitlements, including access to asthma specialists, timely appointments, and comprehensive medication coverage.

5. Seeking communal support: Engaging with asthma support groups, online forums, or community organizations provides opportunities to connect with peers facing similar challenges and share experiences.

Advocating for Others with Asthma

Supporting and advocating for fellow individuals with asthma can significantly enhance their health and well-being:

- **Family support:** Educating family members about asthma management strategies, symptom recognition, and the importance of adherence to treatment plans.

- **Community engagement:** Promoting asthma awareness by disseminating educational materials, organizing community events, or participating in health fairs.

-**School advocacy:** Collaborating with school administrators and educators to ensure asthma action plans are in place for students, medications are readily accessible, and asthma triggers are minimized in educational environments.

- **Workplace initiatives:** Advocating for asthma-friendly workplace environments that include clean air policies, flexible work schedules to accommodate medical appointments, and accessibility to inhalers.

Contributing to Broader Advocacy Efforts

Participation in broader advocacy endeavors contributes to advancing asthma awareness, research, and policy initiatives:

- **Supporting asthma organizations:** Volunteering time, participating in fundraising events, or advocating for policy changes aimed at improving asthma care and increasing research funding.

- **Educating policymakers:** Sharing personal experiences and advocating for policies that prioritize asthma prevention, equitable access to healthcare, and initiatives promoting clean air.

- **Raising public awareness:** Utilizing social media platforms, blogs, or local media outlets to share personal asthma stories, practical tips for managing asthma, and information about upcoming educational resources or events.

-**Engaging in research:** Considering involvement in clinical trials or research studies aimed at advancing scientific knowledge and developing innovative treatment options for asthma.

Addressing Advocacy Challenges

Advocacy efforts for asthma may encounter obstacles such as stigma, resource limitations, or insufficient awareness. Overcoming these challenges involves:

- **Educational initiatives:** Dispelling misconceptions and reducing stigma surrounding asthma through accurate information dissemination.

- **Collaborative efforts:** Partnering with healthcare providers, community organizations, and policymakers to amplify advocacy endeavors and leverage available resources.

- **Persistence and resilience:** Maintaining steadfast commitment to advocating for change despite encountering setbacks or resistance.

Conclusion

Advocacy serves as a potent tool for individuals with asthma to assert their needs, support others within their community, and contribute to initiatives that enhance asthma care and awareness. By advocating for themselves and others, individuals can improve access to quality care, promote education and support, and drive meaningful advancements in asthma management and policy.

In summary, effective advocacy for oneself and others with asthma entails acquiring knowledge, communicating effectively with healthcare providers, maintaining records, understanding rights, seeking support, and actively participating in community and policy initiatives. Through advocacy efforts, individuals with asthma can transcend the limitations imposed by their condition and foster a supportive environment for everyone affected by asthma.

CHAPTER 20: RELIABLE SOURCES FOR MANAGING ASTHMA

Accessing accurate and current information is essential for effectively managing asthma. This chapter explores trustworthy sources that individuals with asthma can use to deepen their understanding, find support, and navigate their healthcare journey.

National Organizations Dedicated to Asthma

National asthma organizations offer a wealth of resources, educational materials, and support networks for individuals living with asthma and their caregivers. These organizations typically provide:

- **Educational resources:** Information on asthma symptoms, triggers, treatments, and strategies for self-management.

- **Support communities:** Online forums, local support groups, or helplines where individuals can connect with others facing similar challenges.

- **Advocacy and policy initiatives:** Opportunities to participate in efforts aimed at improving asthma care, research funding, and public policy.

Examples of National Asthma Organizations:
- **American Lung Association (ALA):** Provides extensive asthma information, educational programs, advocacy opportunities, and support for individuals and families affected by asthma.

- **Asthma and Allergy Foundation of America (AAFA):** Offers resources, educational materials, community support, and advocacy initiatives focused on asthma and allergies.

- **National Asthma Education and Prevention Program (NAEPP):** Established by the National Heart, Lung, and Blood Institute (NHLBI), offers guidelines, research updates, and educational tools for healthcare professionals and individuals with asthma.

Guidance from Healthcare Providers

Healthcare professionals such as primary care physicians, pulmonologists, allergists, and respiratory therapists are invaluable resources for asthma management. They provide:

- **Personalized treatment plans:** Tailored to individual asthma severity, triggers, and lifestyle factors.

-**Education and training:** Guidance on proper inhaler techniques, creating asthma action plans, and strategies for self-monitoring.

- **Regular monitoring:** Scheduled check-ups to assess asthma control, adjust treatment as needed, and address any concerns or complications.

Online Resources and Mobile Applications

In the digital age, numerous online platforms and mobile apps are designed to support asthma management. These resources offer:

- **Educational content:** Articles, videos, and webinars covering asthma symptoms, triggers, medications, and self-care tips.

- **Symptom tracking:** Tools for recording asthma symptoms, peak flow measurements, medication usage, and triggers over time.

- **Medication reminders:** Alerts and notifications to help individuals adhere to prescribed asthma medications and treatment schedules.

Examples of Useful Online Resources and Apps:

- **CDC Asthma:** Provides comprehensive information on asthma management, guidelines, data, and resources for both healthcare providers and individuals with asthma.

- **My Asthma App (by AAFA):** Tracks asthma symptoms, medication usage, triggers, and provides personalized asthma action plans.

- **AsthmaMD:** Offers tools for asthma tracking, symptom monitoring, medication reminders, and personalized reports to share with healthcare providers.

Educational Materials and Publications

Books, pamphlets, and reputable websites dedicated to asthma offer in-depth knowledge and practical advice for managing the condition effectively. These resources include:

- **Comprehensive information:** Detailed insights into asthma symptoms, triggers, treatments, and self-management techniques.

- **Practical tips:** Guidance on lifestyle adjustments, environmental controls, and coping strategies specific to individuals with asthma.

- **Research updates:** Access to the latest advancements in asthma treatment, ongoing clinical trials, and emerging therapies.

Local Community Support

Local community resources are crucial in providing support to individuals with asthma and their families. These resources may include:

- **Community health centers:** Offering asthma education programs, screenings, and access to healthcare services, particularly for underserved populations.

- **Support groups:** Local gatherings where individuals with asthma can share experiences, receive emotional support, and exchange insights on managing their condition.

- School and workplace initiatives: Programs aimed at raising asthma awareness, implementing asthma action plans, and ensuring appropriate accommodations in educational and occupational settings.

Conclusion

Trusted resources for managing asthma empower individuals to navigate their healthcare journey effectively, enhance their knowledge of the condition, and access supportive networks. By utilizing national asthma organizations, seeking guidance from healthcare providers, utilizing online tools and apps, exploring educational materials, and engaging with local community resources, individuals can optimize their asthma management and improve their overall quality of life.

In summary, a combination of reliable information, personalized healthcare guidance, digital tools, educational resources, and local community support forms a robust framework for comprehensive asthma management. By leveraging these trusted resources, individuals with asthma can overcome the challenges posed by their condition and achieve optimal respiratory health.

CHAPTER 21: TIPS FOR TRAVELING WITH ASTHMA

Traveling presents exciting opportunities but requires thorough planning and preparation, particularly for individuals managing asthma. This chapter offers essential advice and strategies to ensure safe and enjoyable travel experiences while effectively managing asthma.

Before You Travel

1. Consult Your Healthcare Provider: Arrange a pre-travel consultation with your healthcare provider, preferably your asthma specialist or primary care physician. Discuss your travel plans, ensure your asthma is well-controlled, and update any necessary vaccinations.

2. Review Your Asthma Action Plan: Confirm your asthma action plan is current. Discuss any adjustments needed for travel, such as changes in medication schedules or coping strategies for different climates.

3. Obtain Sufficient Medications: Pack more than enough asthma medications for your entire trip, including rescue inhalers, maintenance medications, spacers, and any necessary nebulizers. Divide them between your carry-on and checked luggage in case of loss or delays.

4. Research Your Destination: Investigate potential asthma triggers at your destination, such as pollen levels, air quality, altitude, and weather conditions. This information helps you prepare and anticipate challenges.

5. Prepare Travel Documents: Carry copies of your asthma action plan, prescriptions, and a letter from your healthcare provider explaining your medical condition and the necessity of carrying medications and devices.

Packing Essentials

1. Asthma Medications: Pack all medications in their original containers with labels intact. Include extra supply to cover unexpected delays.

2. Allergy Medications: If allergies worsen asthma symptoms (e.g., allergic rhinitis), pack antihistamines or other allergy medications as a precaution.

3. Nebulizer or Spacer: If you use a nebulizer, ensure it is portable. Alternatively, bring a spacer for inhalers to ensure effective medication delivery.

4. Peak Flow Meter: Carry a peak flow meter if regularly used to monitor lung function. It helps assess asthma control during travel.

5. Protective Face Mask: Pack a high-quality face mask to shield against airborne allergens, pollutants, or respiratory infections, especially in crowded or polluted environments.

During Travel

1. Keep Medications Handy: Store asthma medications in your carry-on for quick access during flights or journeys. Avoid placing them in checked luggage to prevent loss or delays.

2. Stay Hydrated: Drink plenty of water to keep airways hydrated, especially in dry or low-humidity environments. Limit caffeine and alcohol intake, which can dehydrate you.

3. Manage Stress: Traveling stress can trigger asthma symptoms. Practice relaxation techniques like deep breathing or meditation to stay calm.

4. Protect against Cold Air: Wear a scarf or face mask in cold climates to warm and humidify the air before breathing it in, reducing the risk of cold-induced asthma symptoms.

5. Monitor Asthma Symptoms: Stay vigilant for changes in asthma symptoms. Use a peak flow meter as needed and follow your action plan for managing flare-ups.

Arriving at Your Destination

1. Check Air Quality: Assess local air quality using resources or apps. Avoid outdoor activities during high pollution or allergen exposure periods.

2. Stay Prepared: Keep asthma medications and supplies organized and accessible throughout your stay. Ensure access to medical care if necessary.

3. Adapt to Climate Changes: Gradually adjust to different climates, as humidity, temperature, and altitude changes can affect asthma symptoms.

4. Communicate Your Needs: Inform travel companions, hotel staff, or guides about your asthma and how they can assist during symptoms or emergencies.

5. Enjoy Your Trip Safely: Despite asthma, plan activities suitable for your health and pace yourself to prevent exhaustion.

Returning Home

1. Review Your Experience: Reflect on travel challenges related to asthma. Note effective strategies and adjustments for future trips.

2. Follow Up with Your Healthcare Provider: Schedule a post-travel appointment to review asthma control and adjust treatment plans as needed.

3. Restock Medications: Ensure an adequate supply of asthma medications for daily use and future travel needs.

4. Share Your Experience: Share travel insights in asthma support groups or forums to assist others preparing for trips.

5. Plan Your Next Adventure: With proper preparation, asthma should not limit travel. Look forward to future trips with confidence and enthusiasm!

Conclusion

Traveling with asthma requires careful planning, proactive management, and awareness of triggers and challenges. By consulting healthcare providers, preparing thoroughly, packing essentials, managing symptoms, adapting to new environments, and reflecting on experiences, individuals with asthma can enjoy safe and fulfilling travel. With these strategies, asthma need not hinder exploration and enjoyment of the world while maintaining optimal respiratory health.

In summary, whether planning a short trip or extended vacation, following these tips for traveling with asthma ensures confident navigation and effective asthma management throughout travels. Proactive steps and readiness enable safe, enjoyable experiences, embracing the wonders of travel while prioritizing respiratory wellness.

CHAPTER 22: DISPELLING MYTHS ABOUT ASTHMA AND ALLERGIES

Asthma and allergies affect millions globally, yet many misconceptions about these conditions persist. These misunderstandings can hinder effective management and create unnecessary challenges for those affected. This chapter aims to debunk common myths about asthma and allergies, providing accurate information to help individuals better manage their conditions.

Myth 1: Asthma Only Affects Children

-**Reality:** Although asthma often starts in childhood, it is not limited to children. Many adults develop asthma later in life, known as adult-onset asthma. Asthma can continue into adulthood for those diagnosed as children, and older adults may develop asthma due to factors like occupational exposures, respiratory infections, or immune system changes. Recognizing that asthma can occur at any age is essential for proper diagnosis and management throughout life.

Myth 2: Exercise Should Be Avoided by Those with Asthma

-**Reality:** Exercise is beneficial for everyone, including people with asthma. Regular physical activity improves cardiovascular health, strengthens the immune system, and enhances overall well-being. While exercise-induced bronchoconstriction (EIB) may be a concern, it can often be managed with pre-exercise medication and appropriate warm-ups. Consulting a healthcare provider for a tailored exercise plan is crucial. Many athletes with asthma successfully compete, showing that asthma should not prevent an active lifestyle.

Myth 3: Asthma Medications Are Addictive

-Reality: Asthma medications, including inhalers, are not addictive. They are vital for controlling symptoms and preventing asthma attacks. Inhaled corticosteroids, commonly used as long-term control medications, reduce airway inflammation and prevent symptoms. These medications are safe when used as prescribed and are crucial for maintaining good asthma control. Worry about dependency should not stop individuals from using their prescribed medications, as proper use can greatly enhance quality of life and prevent severe exacerbations.

Myth 4: Moving to a Different Climate Will Cure Asthma

-**Reality:** Relocating might provide temporary relief for some, but it is not a cure for asthma. Environmental factors such as pollen, pollution, and humidity vary, and what seems beneficial initially may not offer long-term improvement. Asthma is a chronic condition with multiple triggers, and effective management usually involves a combination of medication, lifestyle adjustments, and trigger avoidance, rather than moving to a new location.

Myth 5: Allergies Are Not Serious

-**Reality:** Allergies can range from mild to severe, significantly impacting quality of life. Allergic reactions can cause symptoms like sneezing, itching, and hives, and in severe cases, can lead to anaphylaxis, a potentially life-threatening reaction requiring immediate medical attention. For those with asthma, allergies can worsen symptoms and trigger asthma attacks. Proper diagnosis and management of allergies are crucial to prevent complications and enhance overall health.

Myth 6: Asthma Is Caused by Psychological Factors

-Reality: Asthma is a physical condition characterized by airway inflammation and narrowing, making breathing difficult. While stress and emotions can trigger symptoms, they do not cause asthma. The primary causes of asthma involve a mix of genetic and environmental factors. It is essential to recognize asthma as a physical condition that needs medical management and should not be viewed as a psychological issue.

Myth 7: Asthma Can Be Outgrown

-Reality: Some children may experience a reduction in symptoms or appear to outgrow asthma as they age. However, asthma can return later, and some individuals may have chronic symptoms into adulthood. Asthma is a lifelong condition that can go into remission but may reappear, especially if triggered by environmental factors or respiratory infections. Continuous monitoring and management are needed to keep asthma under control.

Myth 8: Over-the-Counter Medications Are Enough for Asthma Management

-Reality: While over-the-counter (OTC) medications can offer temporary relief for mild allergy symptoms, they are not sufficient for managing asthma. Asthma requires prescription medications to control inflammation and prevent symptoms. Inhaled corticosteroids, long-acting beta-agonists, and leukotriene modifiers are examples of prescription medications used to effectively manage asthma. Relying solely on OTC medications can result in poor asthma control and increased risk of severe attacks.

Myth 9: All Inhalers Are the Same

-Reality: Different types of inhalers are used to manage asthma, each with a specific purpose. Rescue inhalers, like short-acting beta-agonists (SABAs), provide quick relief of acute symptoms. Maintenance inhalers, which may contain corticosteroids or long-acting beta-agonists (LABAs), are used daily to control chronic symptoms and prevent exacerbations. Understanding the differences and using inhalers correctly is vital for effective asthma management.

Myth 10: Asthma Is a Minor Inconvenience

-**Reality:** Asthma is a serious chronic condition that can significantly impact daily life. Without proper management, asthma can lead to frequent hospitalizations, missed school or work days, and reduced quality of life. Severe asthma attacks can be life-threatening. It is crucial to take asthma seriously, follow medical advice, and adhere to prescribed treatment plans to maintain good control and prevent complications.

Conclusion

Dispelling myths about asthma and allergies is crucial for improving understanding, reducing stigma, and promoting effective management. By addressing these misconceptions and providing accurate information, individuals with asthma and allergies can better manage their conditions and achieve a higher quality of life. Proper education and awareness are key to breaking free from the limitations of asthma and allergies, empowering individuals to live healthier, more fulfilling lives.

CHAPTER 23: STRATEGIES TO NAVIGATE THE SEPTEMBER ASTHMA PEAK

As summer ends and September begins, many individuals with asthma notice a significant increase in symptoms. This surge, known as the "September Asthma Peak," is due to several factors, including the return to school, higher exposure to respiratory infections, and seasonal allergen changes. Effectively managing asthma during this period requires a proactive approach and a thorough understanding of the triggers.

This chapter outlines strategies to manage asthma during the September peak, ensuring better control and reducing the risk of exacerbations.

Understanding the September Asthma Peak

The September Asthma Peak is the observed increase in asthma exacerbations during early September. Several factors contribute to this seasonal rise:

1. Return to School: When children and teens go back to school, they are exposed to crowded environments, increasing their chances of contracting viral infections like the common cold, which can trigger asthma symptoms and severe exacerbations.

2. Seasonal Allergens: Fall allergens like ragweed pollen and mold spores become more prevalent, worsening asthma symptoms for those sensitive to these allergens.

3. Weather Changes: The transition from summer to fall brings fluctuations in temperature and humidity, which can irritate the airways and trigger asthma symptoms.

4. Reduced Medication Adherence: Some individuals may become less diligent with their asthma management routines over the summer, leading to decreased adherence to prescribed medications and increased vulnerability to triggers.

Strategies for Managing the September Asthma Peak

Managing asthma during the September peak requires a multifaceted approach. The following strategies can help individuals navigate this challenging period:

1. Maintain Consistent Medication Adherence

Adherence to prescribed medications is crucial for asthma management. Ensure that you:

- Continue Daily Controller Medications: Even if symptoms improve during the summer, it is essential to continue using daily controller medications as prescribed. These medications, like inhaled corticosteroids, help reduce airway inflammation and prevent exacerbations.

- Use Rescue Inhalers Appropriately: Always carry a rescue inhaler (such as albuterol) to manage acute symptoms. Use it as directed by your healthcare provider.

- Review Medication Plans with Your Doctor: Before the school year starts, schedule an appointment with your healthcare provider to review and update your asthma action plan. Ensure your medication regimen is optimized for the upcoming season.

2. Minimize Exposure to Allergens

Reducing exposure to allergens can significantly improve asthma control. Consider these measures:

- Monitor Pollen Counts: Stay informed about daily pollen counts and try to limit outdoor activities during peak pollen times, usually in the early morning and late afternoon.

- Use Air Purifiers: Invest in air purifiers with HEPA filters to help reduce indoor allergen levels, such as pollen and mold spores.

- Keep Windows Closed: During high pollen days, keep windows and doors closed to prevent allergens from entering your home.

- Clean Regularly: Regularly clean your living spaces to minimize dust and mold accumulation. Use a damp cloth for dusting and vacuum with a HEPA filter vacuum cleaner.

3. Strengthen Immune Defense

Building a robust immune system can help reduce the risk of respiratory infections that can trigger asthma symptoms. Focus on the following:

- Maintain a Balanced Diet: Consume a diet rich in fruits, vegetables, lean proteins, and whole grains to support overall health and immunity.

- Stay Hydrated: Drink plenty of water to keep your airways hydrated and help your body fight off infections.

- Get Adequate Sleep: Ensure you get sufficient rest, as sleep is crucial for a healthy immune system.

- Exercise Regularly: Engage in regular physical activity to boost your immune system. Be mindful of exercise-induced asthma and take necessary precautions, such as using pre-exercise medication if needed.

4. Implement Hygiene Practices

Good hygiene practices can help prevent the spread of respiratory infections, particularly in school settings:

- Teach Proper Handwashing: Encourage frequent handwashing with soap and water, especially after coughing, sneezing, or touching shared surfaces.

- Use Hand Sanitizers: When soap and water are not available, use hand sanitizers with at least 60% alcohol.

- Avoid Close Contact with Sick Individuals: Try to minimize close contact with individuals who are showing symptoms of respiratory infections.

- Teach Coughing and Sneezing Etiquette: Encourage coughing or sneezing into a tissue or the elbow to prevent the spread of germs.

5. Plan for School

For children and adolescents with asthma, returning to school can be particularly challenging. The following steps can help ensure a smooth transition:

- Inform School Staff: Ensure teachers, school nurses, and administrators are aware of your child's asthma condition and have a copy of their asthma action plan.

- Provide Necessary Medications: Ensure your child has access to their asthma medications at school, including a rescue inhaler. Check that all medications are up-to-date and that the school has clear instructions for their use.

- Educate Your Child: Teach your child to recognize asthma symptoms and understand how to use their medications properly. Empower them to communicate with teachers and school staff if they feel unwell.

Conclusion

The September Asthma Peak presents a unique set of challenges for individuals with asthma. By understanding the contributing factors and implementing proactive strategies, it is possible to navigate this period with greater ease and control. Consistent medication adherence, minimizing allergen exposure, strengthening immune defenses, practicing good hygiene, and planning for school are all critical components of effective asthma management. With these strategies in place, individuals with asthma can better manage their condition, reduce the risk of exacerbations, and enjoy a healthier, more active life.

LAST CHAPTER: COMMON QUESTIONS ASKED BY PATIENTS AND THEIR ANSWERS

Managing asthma often leads to many questions about the condition, treatment options, and necessary lifestyle changes. Addressing these questions thoroughly can significantly enhance a patient's ability to effectively manage their asthma. In this final chapter, we will delve into some of the most commonly asked questions by asthma patients and provide clear, informative answers to guide you on your path to better asthma management.

What is Asthma?

Asthma is a chronic respiratory condition marked by inflammation and narrowing of the airways, leading to breathing difficulties, coughing, wheezing, and shortness of breath. The severity of asthma can range from mild to severe, and it can be triggered by various factors, including allergens, respiratory infections, exercise, and environmental pollutants.

What Causes Asthma?

The exact cause of asthma remains unclear, but it is believed to stem from a mix of genetic and environmental factors. Common triggers include:

- Allergens: Such as pollen, mold, pet dander, and dust mites.
- Respiratory Infections: Like colds, flu, and other viral infections.
- Irritants: Including smoke, pollution, strong odors, and chemical fumes.
- Exercise: Physical activity can trigger symptoms, known as exercise-induced asthma.
- Weather Changes: Fluctuations in temperature and humidity can provoke symptoms.

- Stress: Emotional stress and anxiety can aggravate asthma symptoms.

How is Asthma Diagnosed?

Asthma is usually diagnosed through a combination of medical history, physical examination, and lung function tests. Key diagnostic tools include:

- Spirometry: Measures the amount of air you can exhale and the speed at which you can do so.
- Peak Flow Meter: A simple device to assess how well your lungs are functioning.

- Allergy Testing: Identifies specific allergens that may be triggering your asthma.

What are the Different Types of Asthma?

Asthma comes in various forms, each with unique characteristics:

- Allergic Asthma: Triggered by allergens like pollen, mold, and pet dander.
- Non-Allergic Asthma: Triggered by irritants such as smoke, pollution, and strong odors.
- Exercise-Induced Asthma: Triggered by physical activity.

- Occupational Asthma: Triggered by exposure to substances in the workplace.
- Nocturnal Asthma: Symptoms worsen at night, disrupting sleep.

How Can Asthma be Managed?

Effective asthma management involves medication, lifestyle changes, and regular monitoring. Key components include:

- Medication: Asthma medications are typically divided into two categories:
  - Controller Medications: Used daily to reduce inflammation and prevent symptoms, such as inhaled

corticosteroids and long-acting beta-agonists.

   - Rescue Medications: Used to provide quick relief during an asthma attack, such as short-acting beta-agonists like albuterol.

- Asthma Action Plan: A personalized plan developed with your healthcare provider to manage your asthma, including information on daily management, recognizing worsening symptoms, and emergency actions.

- Avoiding Triggers: Identifying and minimizing exposure to asthma triggers.

- Regular Monitoring: Using devices like peak flow meters to monitor lung function and track symptoms.

Can Asthma be Cured?

While there is no cure for asthma, it can be effectively managed with appropriate treatment and lifestyle adjustments. Many people with asthma lead normal, active lives by following their asthma action plan and taking their medications as prescribed.

What Should I Do During an Asthma Attack?

During an asthma attack, it is crucial to act quickly to prevent symptoms from worsening. Follow these steps:

1. Stay Calm: Anxiety can worsen symptoms, so try to remain calm.
2. Use Your Rescue Inhaler: Take the prescribed number of puffs from your rescue inhaler. If symptoms do not improve, follow the instructions in your asthma action plan.
3. Seek Medical Help if Needed: If symptoms do not improve or worsen after using your rescue inhaler, seek emergency medical assistance immediately.

How Can I Improve My Quality of Life with Asthma?

Improving your quality of life with asthma involves proactive management and healthy lifestyle choices. Consider these tips:

- Stay Active: Engage in regular physical activity that is suitable for your condition. Consult your healthcare provider about pre-exercise medications if needed.
- Healthy Diet: Eat a balanced diet rich in fruits, vegetables, lean proteins, and whole grains to support overall health and immune function.

- Quit Smoking: If you smoke, seek help to quit. Avoid exposure to secondhand smoke and other environmental pollutants.
- Manage Stress: Practice stress-reducing techniques such as yoga, meditation, and deep-breathing exercises.
- Regular Check-Ups: Schedule regular appointments with your healthcare provider to monitor your condition and adjust your treatment plan as necessary.

What Should I Know About Asthma in Children?

Asthma in children requires careful management and monitoring. Parents and caregivers should:

- Understand Triggers: Identify and minimize exposure to your child's asthma triggers.
- Medication Adherence: Ensure your child takes their asthma medications as prescribed.
- Education: Teach your child about their condition and how to manage it. Ensure they know how to use their inhaler correctly.

- School Communication: Inform teachers, school nurses, and other relevant staff about your child's asthma and provide them with a copy of the asthma action plan.
- Emergency Preparedness: Ensure your child has access to their rescue inhaler at all times, including at school and during extracurricular activities.

What Resources are Available for Asthma Patients?

Numerous resources are available to support asthma patients:

- Healthcare Providers: Your primary care physician, pulmonologist, and

asthma specialist can provide personalized care and guidance.
- Asthma Support Groups: Joining a support group can provide emotional support and practical tips from others living with asthma.
- Educational Materials: Many organizations offer educational resources, including brochures, videos, and online courses, to help you better understand and manage your asthma.
- Mobile Apps: There are various apps available that can help you track your symptoms, medication use, and lung function.

Conclusion

Living with asthma can be challenging, but with the right knowledge and tools, you can take control of your condition and lead a fulfilling life. By understanding your asthma, adhering to your treatment plan, avoiding triggers, and making healthy lifestyle choices, you can effectively manage your symptoms and reduce the risk of exacerbations. Remember to work closely with your healthcare provider, stay informed, and seek support when needed. With dedication and proactive management, you can break free from the limitations of asthma and enjoy a healthier, more active life.

Vote of Thanks

As we conclude "Breaking Free from Asthma! Your Essential Guide to Managing and Overcoming Respiratory Challenges," we extend our heartfelt gratitude to everyone who contributed to the creation of this ebook.

Firstly, a sincere thank you to our readers. Your dedication to learning and proactive approach to managing asthma have been the driving force behind this project. We hope the insights and strategies in this book empower you to take control of your asthma and live a healthier, more fulfilling life.

We are immensely grateful to the healthcare professionals who shared their knowledge and experiences. Your contributions have been invaluable in shaping the content, ensuring its accuracy and practicality. Special thanks to the doctors, pulmonologists, nurses, and respiratory therapists who provided their expertise and reviewed the material to ensure its medical reliability.

A special acknowledgment goes to the asthma patients and their families who shared their personal stories. Your bravery, resilience, and openness have added a deeply personal and relatable aspect to this ebook, offering hope and inspiration to others facing similar challenges.

We also want to recognize the researchers and scientists whose relentless work in the field of asthma has led to better treatments and a deeper understanding of this condition. Your commitment to advancing medical knowledge and developing innovative therapies continues to significantly impact the lives of those living with asthma.

To our editorial team, thank you for your dedication and meticulous attention to detail. Your efforts in organizing, editing, and refining the content have ensured this ebook is a comprehensive and accessible guide for our readers.

Special thanks to the designers and technical experts who worked behind the scenes to create an engaging and user-friendly ebook. Your creativity and technical skills have made it possible to present the information in a visually appealing and easily navigable format.

Lastly, we express our gratitude to the organizations and institutions that provided support and resources for this project. Your collaboration and support have been crucial in bringing this ebook to life.

As you finish reading "Breaking Free from Asthma!", we hope it serves as a valuable resource in your journey toward better asthma management. We would greatly appreciate your thoughts and feedback. Please take a moment to leave a review on Amazon. Your reviews not only help us improve future editions but also assist others in discovering this book and benefiting from its insights.

Thank you once again for being a part of this endeavor. Together, we can continue to overcome the challenges of asthma and strive for a healthier, more active life.

With sincere appreciation,

Louis Baker

Printed in Great Britain
by Amazon